ATS-99   ADMISSION TEST SERIES

This is your
PASSBOOK for...

Allied Health Professions Admission Test (AHPAT)

Test Preparation Study Guide
Questions & Answers

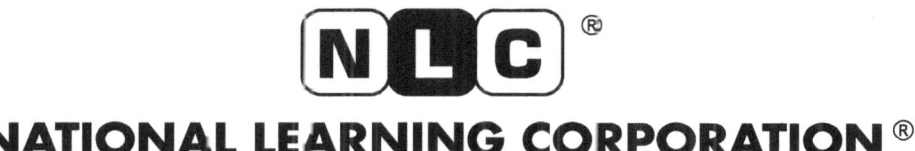

COPYRIGHT NOTICE

This book is SOLELY intended for, is sold ONLY to, and its use is RESTRICTED to individual, bona fide applicants or candidates who qualify by virtue of having seriously filed applications for appropriate license, certificate, professional and/or promotional advancement, higher school matriculation, scholarship, or other legitimate requirements of education and/or governmental authorities.

This book is NOT intended for use, class instruction, tutoring, training, duplication, copying, reprinting, excerption, or adaptation, etc., by:

1) Other publishers
2) Proprietors and/or Instructors of "Coaching" and/or Preparatory Courses
3) Personnel and/or Training Divisions of commercial, industrial, and governmental organizations
4) Schools, colleges, or universities and/or their departments and staffs, including teachers and other personnel
5) Testing Agencies or Bureaus
6) Study groups which seek by the purchase of a single volume to copy and/or duplicate and/or adapt this material for use by the group as a whole without having purchased individual volumes for each of the members of the group
7) Et al.

Such persons would be in violation of appropriate Federal and State statutes.

PROVISION OF LICENSING AGREEMENTS – Recognized educational, commercial, industrial, and governmental institutions and organizations, and others legitimately engaged in educational pursuits, including training, testing, and measurement activities, may address request for a licensing agreement to the copyright owners, who will determine whether, and under what conditions, including fees and charges, the materials in this book may be used them. In other words, a licensing facility exists for the legitimate use of the material in this book on other than an individual basis. However, it is asseverated and affirmed here that the material in this book CANNOT be used without the receipt of the express permission of such a licensing agreement from the Publishers. Inquiries re licensing should be addressed to the company, attention rights and permissions department.

All rights reserved, including the right of reproduction in whole or in part, in any form or by any means, electronic or mechanical, including photocopying, recording, or by any information storage and retrieval system, without permission in writing from the Publisher.

Copyright © 2024 by
National Learning Corporation

212 Michael Drive, Syosset, NY 11791
(516) 921-8888 • www.passbooks.com
E-mail: info@passbooks.com

PUBLISHED IN THE UNITED STATES OF AMERICA

PASSBOOK® SERIES

THE *PASSBOOK® SERIES* has been created to prepare applicants and candidates for the ultimate academic battlefield – the examination room.

At some time in our lives, each and every one of us may be required to take an examination – for validation, matriculation, admission, qualification, registration, certification, or licensure.

Based on the assumption that every applicant or candidate has met the basic formal educational standards, has taken the required number of courses, and read the necessary texts, the *PASSBOOK® SERIES* furnishes the one special preparation which may assure passing with confidence, instead of failing with insecurity. Examination questions – together with answers – are furnished as the basic vehicle for study so that the mysteries of the examination and its compounding difficulties may be eliminated or diminished by a sure method.

This book is meant to help you pass your examination provided that you qualify and are serious in your objective.

The entire field is reviewed through the huge store of content information which is succinctly presented through a provocative and challenging approach – the question-and-answer method.

A climate of success is established by furnishing the correct answers at the end of each test.

You soon learn to recognize types of questions, forms of questions, and patterns of questioning. You may even begin to anticipate expected outcomes.

You perceive that many questions are repeated or adapted so that you can gain acute insights, which may enable you to score many sure points.

You learn how to confront new questions, or types of questions, and to attack them confidently and work out the correct answers.

You note objectives and emphases, and recognize pitfalls and dangers, so that you may make positive educational adjustments.

Moreover, you are kept fully informed in relation to new concepts, methods, practices, and directions in the field.

You discover that you are actually taking the examination all the time: you are preparing for the examination by "taking" an examination, not by reading extraneous and/or supererogatory textbooks.

In short, this PASSBOOK®, used directedly, should be an important factor in helping you to pass your test.

Allied Health Professions Admission Test

AHPAT

All correspondence and requests for information concerning the Allied Health Professions Admission Test (AHPAT) should be directed to:

Allied Health Professions Admission Test
The Psychological Corporation
555 Academic Court
San Antonio, Texas 78204
(512) 921-8794

GENERAL INFORMATION

The Allied Health Professions Admission Test is prepared and administered by The Psychological Corporation for applicants seeking admission to baccalaureate and post-baccalaureate programs in allied health schools. It is designed to measure general academic ability and scientific knowledge. The extent to which test results are used in deciding whether or not an applicant will be admitted to a school of allied health varies from one school to another. In general, test results are combined with other information, such as high school and undergraduate records, references and results of personal interviews.

Results are sent to the examinee and schools of allied health approximately **four weeks** following the date of testing.

By submitting their Applications, applicants agree to be bound by the procedures and policies set forth in this Announcement.

Whenever you call The Psychological Corporation, you should keep a record of when you called, the name of the person you spoke to, and the information you were given. It is a good practice to follow up any telephone conversation with a letter.

CONTENT OF TEST

The AHPAT is a specialized test to help identify qualified students planning to enter allied health professions. The content of each test is carefully prepared to predict an applicant's academic ability to complete professional studies in allied health. The test is so designed that no examinee is expected to answer all the questions correctly. Scores are based on the number of correct answers only; there is no penalty for "guessing" as such. The AHPAT measures abilities in the following areas:

Verbal Ability - A test of general vocabulary and verbal reasoning.

Quantitative Ability - A measure of ability to reason through and understand quantitative concepts and relationships.

Biology - Survey of principles and concepts in basic biology with major emphasis on human biology.

Chemistry - Sampling of problems and principles in elementary college chemistry.

Reading Comprehension - Ability to read and understand written materials in textbook style; reading passages and questions primarily science-oriented.

The Psychological Corporation does not publish any study materials for this test and does not recommend any specific study materials.

SAMPLE QUESTIONS

All the questions in the test are of the objective, multiple-choice type. Answers will be marked on separate answer sheets. You should take several sharpened Number 2 pencils with erasers to the Testing Center. The following sample questions are illustrative of those found in the examination. Correct answers to these questions are indicated on page **2**.

Verbal Ability
Directions: Choose the word which means the SAME or most nearly the same as the word in capitals.

1. APPEND
   A. Reduce
   B. Attach
   C. Oppose
   D. Request

2. CRYPTIC
   A. Deadly
   B. Obscure
   C. Sarcastic
   D. Overwhelming

Directions: Choose the word which means the OPPOSITE or most nearly opposite to the word in capitals.

3. SOLEMN
   A. Jolly
   B. Overt
   C. Willful
   D. Infamous

4. HINDER
   A. Erect
   B. Advise
   C. Simplify
   D. Further

Quantitative Ability
Directions: Choose the one best answer to each of the following questions.

5. $1 \frac{2}{3} + 3 \frac{1}{6} + 2 \frac{1}{3} =$
   A. $6 \frac{1}{6}$
   B. $6 \frac{2}{3}$
   C. $7 \frac{1}{6}$
   D. $7 \frac{1}{3}$

6. If a colony of 200 bacteria doubles its numbers every 6 hours, how many bacteria will there be at the end of a day?
   A. 400
   B. 800
   C. 1600
   D. 3200

7. If the radius of a circle is halved, by how much does the circumference decrease?
   A. 10%
   B. 25%
   C. 33 1/3%
   D. 50%

8. .36 is what percent of .144?
   A. 25%
   B. 40%
   C. 250%
   D. 400%

Biology
Directions: Choose the best answer to each of the following questions.

9. RNA and DNA are alike in that both
   A. contain uracil.
   B. contain deoxyribose.
   C. are double-stranded.
   D. have codons consisting of 3 nucleotides.

10. The hormone usually secreted when an animal senses danger and which causes the "fight or flight" reaction is
    A. insulin.
    B. thyroxine.
    C. adrenaline.
    D. parathormone.

11. In which of the following parts of the human circulatory system would the blood pressure be at its lowest level?
    A. In the aorta
    B. In the arterioles
    C. In the pulmonary artery
    D. In the posterior vena cava

Chemistry
Directions: Choose the best answer to each of the following questions.

12. If a mixture of 70% oxygen and 30% hydrogen exerts a total pressure of 700 mm of mercury, then the oxygen exerts a partial pressure of
    A. 210 mm.
    B. 350 mm.
    C. 490 mm.
    D. 700 mm.

13. Isotopes of the same element differ with respect to
    A. mass numbers.
    B. atomic numbers.
    C. electron configuration.
    D. number of protons in the nucleus.

14. What is the oxidation number of bromine in mercury II bromate, $Hg(BrO_3)_2$?
    A. −1
    B. +1
    C. +3
    D. +5

Reading Comprehension
Directions: Read the following passage and then choose the one best answer to each of the questions following the passage.

Cirrhosis is the term applied to the end stage of scarring of the liver. It may follow repeated minor insults or a sudden massive injury. The more common causes are nutritional deficiency, viral infections, injury by chemical agents (postnecrotic cirrhosis), obstruction of the drainage of bile from the liver (biliary cirrhosis), and prolonged and severe heart failure (congestive or cardiac cirrhosis). Since the use of antibiotics, syphilis has become relatively uncommon as a cause of cirrhosis. Because the liver has a large functional reserve, minor degrees of cirrhosis have little physiological effect. Tumors of the nonmalignant type are rare in the liver except for the neoplasm of blood vessels called hemangiomas. These, as well as less common benign tumors of the liver, are usually small and of little significance. Malignant tumors of the liver appear to be increasing in frequency. They are not amenable to surgical treatment and are rapidly fatal. Such tumors usually arise from the liver cells themselves (hepatomas) or from the bile ducts within the liver (cholangiomas). They are particularly common in livers with portal or postnecrotic cirrhosis.

15. The word *insults* as used in the passage means
    A. scorns.
    B. outrages.
    C. assaults.
    D. rudeness.

16. Hepatomas and cholangiomas most frequently occur in people whose livers have been injured by
    A. parasites.
    B. chemical agents.
    C. syphilitic germs.
    D. severe heart failure.

17. What is a hemangioma?
    A. A benign tumor of the liver
    B. A form of biliary cirrhosis
    C. A malignant tumor of the liver
    D. A rupture of the blood vessels in the liver

18. Antibiotics have reduced the incidence of cirrhosis of the liver that is caused by
    A. viruses.
    B. syphilis.
    C. severe heart failure.
    D. obstruction of the bile duct.

CORRECT ANSWERS

1. B 2. B 3. A 4. D 5. C 6. D 7. D
8. C 9. D 10. C 11. D 12. C 13. A
14. D 15. C 16. B 17. A 18. B

HOW TO TAKE A TEST

You have studied long, hard and conscientiously.

With your official admission card in hand, and your heart pounding, you have been admitted to the examination room.

You note that there are several hundred other applicants in the examination room waiting to take the same test.

They all appear to be equally well prepared.

You know that nothing but your best effort will suffice. The "moment of truth" is at hand: you now have to demonstrate objectively, in writing, your knowledge of content and your understanding of subject matter.

You are fighting the most important battle of your life—to pass and/or score high on an examination which will determine your career and provide the economic basis for your livelihood.

What extra, special things should you know and should you do in taking the examination?

I. YOU MUST PASS AN EXAMINATION

A. WHAT EVERY CANDIDATE SHOULD KNOW
  Examination applicants often ask us for help in preparing for the written test. What can I study in advance? What kinds of questions will be asked? How will the test be given? How will the papers be graded?

B. HOW ARE EXAMS DEVELOPED?
  Examinations are carefully written by trained technicians who are specialists in the field known as "psychological measurement," in consultation with recognized authorities in the field of work that the test will cover. These experts recommend the subject matter areas or skills to be tested; only those knowledges or skills important to your success on the job are included. The most reliable books and source materials available are used as references. Together, the experts and technicians judge the difficulty level of the questions.
  Test technicians know how to phrase questions so that the problem is clearly stated. Their ethics do not permit "trick" or "catch" questions. Questions may have been tried out on sample groups, or subjected to statistical analysis, to determine their usefulness.
  Written tests are often used in combination with performance tests, ratings of training and experience, and oral interviews. All of these measures combine to form the best-known means of finding the right person for the right job.

II. HOW TO PASS THE WRITTEN TEST

A. BASIC STEPS

1) Study the announcement

How, then, can you know what subjects to study? Our best answer is: "Learn as much as possible about the class of positions for which you've applied." The exam will test the knowledge, skills and abilities needed to do the work.

Your most valuable source of information about the position you want is the official exam announcement. This announcement lists the training and experience qualifications. Check these standards and apply only if you come reasonably close to meeting them. Many jurisdictions preview the written test in the exam announcement by including a section called "Knowledge and Abilities Required," "Scope of the Examination," or some similar heading. Here you will find out specifically what fields will be tested.

2) Choose appropriate study materials

If the position for which you are applying is technical or advanced, you will read more advanced, specialized material. If you are already familiar with the basic principles of your field, elementary textbooks would waste your time. Concentrate on advanced textbooks and technical periodicals. Think through the concepts and review difficult problems in your field.

These are all general sources. You can get more ideas on your own initiative, following these leads. For example, training manuals and publications of the government agency which employs workers in your field can be useful, particularly for technical and professional positions. A letter or visit to the government department involved may result in more specific study suggestions, and certainly will provide you with a more definite idea of the exact nature of the position you are seeking.

3) Study this book!

III. KINDS OF TESTS

Tests are used for purposes other than measuring knowledge and ability to perform specified duties. For some positions, it is equally important to test ability to make adjustments to new situations or to profit from training. In others, basic mental abilities not dependent on information are essential. Questions which test these things may not appear as pertinent to the duties of the position as those which test for knowledge and information. Yet they are often highly important parts of a fair examination. For very general questions, it is almost impossible to help you direct your study efforts. What we can do is to point out some of the more common of these general abilities needed in public service positions and describe some typical questions.

1) General information

Broad, general information has been found useful for predicting job success in some kinds of work. This is tested in a variety of ways, from vocabulary lists to questions about current events. Basic background in some field of work, such as sociology or economics, may be sampled in a group of questions. Often these are principles which have become familiar to most persons through exposure rather than through formal training. It is difficult to advise you how to study for these questions; being alert to the world around you is our best suggestion.

2) Verbal ability

An example of an ability needed in many positions is verbal or language ability. Verbal ability is, in brief, the ability to use and understand words. Vocabulary and grammar tests are typical measures of this ability. Reading comprehension or paragraph interpretation questions are common in many kinds of civil service tests. You are given a paragraph of written material and asked to find its central meaning.

IV. KINDS OF QUESTIONS

1. Multiple-choice Questions

Most popular of the short-answer questions is the "multiple choice" or "best answer" question. It can be used, for example, to test for factual knowledge, ability to solve problems or judgment in meeting situations found at work.

A multiple-choice question is normally one of three types:
- It can begin with an incomplete statement followed by several possible endings. You are to find the one ending which best completes the statement, although some of the others may not be entirely wrong.
- It can also be a complete statement in the form of a question which is answered by choosing one of the statements listed.
- It can be in the form of a problem – again you select the best answer.

Here is an example of a multiple-choice question with a discussion which should give you some clues as to the method for choosing the right answer:

When an employee has a complaint about his assignment, the action which will best help him overcome his difficulty is to
- A. discuss his difficulty with his coworkers
- B. take the problem to the head of the organization
- C. take the problem to the person who gave him the assignment
- D. say nothing to anyone about his complaint

In answering this question, you should study each of the choices to find which is best. Consider choice "A" – Certainly an employee may discuss his complaint with fellow employees, but no change or improvement can result, and the complaint remains unresolved. Choice "B" is a poor choice since the head of the organization probably does not know what assignment you have been given, and taking your problem to him is known as "going over the head" of the supervisor. The supervisor, or person who made the assignment, is the person who can clarify it or correct any injustice. Choice "C" is, therefore, correct. To say nothing, as in choice "D," is unwise. Supervisors have and interest in knowing the problems employees are facing, and the employee is seeking a solution to his problem.

2. True/False

3. Matching Questions

Matching an answer from a column of choices within another column.

V. RECORDING YOUR ANSWERS

Computer terminals are used more and more today for many different kinds of exams.

For an examination with very few applicants, you may be told to record your answers in the test booklet itself. Separate answer sheets are much more common. If this separate answer sheet is to be scored by machine – and this is often the case – it is highly important that you mark your answers correctly in order to get credit.

VI. BEFORE THE TEST

YOUR PHYSICAL CONDITION IS IMPORTANT

If you are not well, you can't do your best work on tests. If you are half asleep, you can't do your best either. Here are some tips:

1) Get about the same amount of sleep you usually get. Don't stay up all night before the test, either partying or worrying—DON'T DO IT!
2) If you wear glasses, be sure to wear them when you go to take the test. This goes for hearing aids, too.
3) If you have any physical problems that may keep you from doing your best, be sure to tell the person giving the test. If you are sick or in poor health, you relay cannot do your best on any test. You can always come back and take the test some other time.

Common sense will help you find procedures to follow to get ready for an examination. Too many of us, however, overlook these sensible measures. Indeed, nervousness and fatigue have been found to be the most serious reasons why applicants fail to do their best on civil service tests. Here is a list of reminders:

- Begin your preparation early – Don't wait until the last minute to go scurrying around for books and materials or to find out what the position is all about.
- Prepare continuously – An hour a night for a week is better than an all-night cram session. This has been definitely established. What is more, a night a week for a month will return better dividends than crowding your study into a shorter period of time.
- Locate the place of the exam – You have been sent a notice telling you when and where to report for the examination. If the location is in a different town or otherwise unfamiliar to you, it would be well to inquire the best route and learn something about the building.
- Relax the night before the test – Allow your mind to rest. Do not study at all that night. Plan some mild recreation or diversion; then go to bed early and get a good night's sleep.
- Get up early enough to make a leisurely trip to the place for the test – This way unforeseen events, traffic snarls, unfamiliar buildings, etc. will not upset you.
- Dress comfortably – A written test is not a fashion show. You will be known by number and not by name, so wear something comfortable.
- Leave excess paraphernalia at home – Shopping bags and odd bundles will get in your way. You need bring only the items mentioned in the official notice you received; usually everything you need is provided. Do not bring reference books to the exam. They will only confuse those last minutes and be taken away from you when in the test room.

- Arrive somewhat ahead of time – If because of transportation schedules you must get there very early, bring a newspaper or magazine to take your mind off yourself while waiting.
- Locate the examination room – When you have found the proper room, you will be directed to the seat or part of the room where you will sit. Sometimes you are given a sheet of instructions to read while you are waiting. Do not fill out any forms until you are told to do so; just read them and be prepared.
- Relax and prepare to listen to the instructions
- If you have any physical problem that may keep you from doing your best, be sure to tell the test administrator. If you are sick or in poor health, you really cannot do your best on the exam. You can come back and take the test some other time.

VII. AT THE TEST

The day of the test is here and you have the test booklet in your hand. The temptation to get going is very strong. Caution! There is more to success than knowing the right answers. You must know how to identify your papers and understand variations in the type of short-answer question used in this particular examination. Follow these suggestions for maximum results from your efforts:

1) Cooperate with the monitor

The test administrator has a duty to create a situation in which you can be as much at ease as possible. He will give instructions, tell you when to begin, check to see that you are marking your answer sheet correctly, and so on. He is not there to guard you, although he will see that your competitors do not take unfair advantage. He wants to help you do your best.

2) Listen to all instructions

Don't jump the gun! Wait until you understand all directions. In most civil service tests you get more time than you need to answer the questions. So don't be in a hurry. Read each word of instructions until you clearly understand the meaning. Study the examples, listen to all announcements and follow directions. Ask questions if you do not understand what to do.

3) Identify your papers

Civil service exams are usually identified by number only. You will be assigned a number; you must not put your name on your test papers. Be sure to copy your number correctly. Since more than one exam may be given, copy your exact examination title.

4) Plan your time

Unless you are told that a test is a "speed" or "rate of work" test, speed itself is usually not important. Time enough to answer all the questions will be provided, but this does not mean that you have all day. An overall time limit has been set. Divide the total time (in minutes) by the number of questions to determine the approximate time you have for each question.

5) Do not linger over difficult questions

If you come across a difficult question, mark it with a paper clip (useful to have along) and come back to it when you have been through the booklet. One caution if you do this – be sure to skip a number on your answer sheet as well. Check often to be sure that you have not lost your place and that you are marking in the row numbered the same as the question you are answering.

6) Read the questions
   Be sure you know what the question asks! Many capable people are unsuccessful because they failed to read the questions correctly.

7) Answer all questions
   Unless you have been instructed that a penalty will be deducted for incorrect answers, it is better to guess than to omit a question.

8) Speed tests
   It is often better NOT to guess on speed tests. It has been found that on timed tests people are tempted to spend the last few seconds before time is called in marking answers at random – without even reading them – in the hope of picking up a few extra points. To discourage this practice, the instructions may warn you that your score will be "corrected" for guessing. That is, a penalty will be applied. The incorrect answers will be deducted from the correct ones, or some other penalty formula will be used.

9) Review your answers
   If you finish before time is called, go back to the questions you guessed or omitted to give them further thought. Review other answers if you have time.

10) Return your test materials
    If you are ready to leave before others have finished or time is called, take ALL your materials to the monitor and leave quietly. Never take any test material with you. The monitor can discover whose papers are not complete, and taking a test booklet may be grounds for disqualification.

VIII. EXAMINATION TECHNIQUES

1) Read the general instructions carefully. These are usually printed on the first page of the exam booklet. As a rule, these instructions refer to the timing of the examination; the fact that you should not start work until the signal and must stop work at a signal, etc. If there are any special instructions, such as a choice of questions to be answered, make sure that you note this instruction carefully.

2) When you are ready to start work on the examination, that is as soon as the signal has been given, read the instructions to each question booklet, underline any key words or phrases, such as least, best, outline, describe and the like. In this way you will tend to answer as requested rather than discover on reviewing your paper that you listed without describing, that you selected the worst choice rather than the best choice, etc.

3) If the examination is of the objective or multiple-choice type – that is, each question will also give a series of possible answers: A, B, C or D, and you are called upon to select the best answer and write the letter next to that answer on your answer paper – it is advisable to start answering each question in turn. There may be anywhere from 50 to 100 such questions in the three or four hours allotted and you can see how much time would be taken if you read through all the questions before beginning to answer any. Furthermore, if you

come across a question or group of questions which you know would be difficult to answer, it would undoubtedly affect your handling of all the other questions.

4) If the examination is of the essay type and contains but a few questions, it is a moot point as to whether you should read all the questions before starting to answer any one. Of course, if you are given a choice – say five out of seven and the like – then it is essential to read all the questions so you can eliminate the two that are most difficult. If, however, you are asked to answer all the questions, there may be danger in trying to answer the easiest one first because you may find that you will spend too much time on it. The best technique is to answer the first question, then proceed to the second, etc.

5) Time your answers. Before the exam begins, write down the time it started, then add the time allowed for the examination and write down the time it must be completed, then divide the time available somewhat as follows:
   - If 3-1/2 hours are allowed, that would be 210 minutes. If you have 80 objective-type questions, that would be an average of 2-1/2 minutes per question. Allow yourself no more than 2 minutes per question, or a total of 160 minutes, which will permit about 50 minutes to review.
   - If for the time allotment of 210 minutes there are 7 essay questions to answer, that would average about 30 minutes a question. Give yourself only 25 minutes per question so that you have about 35 minutes to review.

6) The most important instruction is to read each question and make sure you know what is wanted. The second most important instruction is to time yourself properly so that you answer every question. The third most important instruction is to answer every question. Guess if you have to but include something for each question. Remember that you will receive no credit for a blank and will probably receive some credit if you write something in answer to an essay question. If you guess a letter – say "B" for a multiple-choice question – you may have guessed right. If you leave a blank as an answer to a multiple-choice question, the examiners may respect your feelings but it will not add a point to your score. Some exams may penalize you for wrong answers, so in such cases only, you may not want to guess unless you have some basis for your answer.

7) Suggestions
   a. Objective-type questions
      1. Examine the question booklet for proper sequence of pages and questions
      2. Read all instructions carefully
      3. Skip any question which seems too difficult; return to it after all other questions have been answered
      4. Apportion your time properly; do not spend too much time on any single question or group of questions
      5. Note and underline key words – all, most, fewest, least, best, worst, same, opposite, etc.
      6. Pay particular attention to negatives
      7. Note unusual option e.g., unduly long, short, complex, different or similar in content to the body of the question
      8. Observe the use of "hedging" words – probably, may, most likely, etc.

9. Make sure that your answer is put next to the same number as the question
10. Do not second-guess unless you have good reason to believe the second answer is definitely more correct
11. Cross out original answer if you decide another answer is more accurate; do not erase until you are ready to hand your paper in
12. Answer all questions; guess unless instructed otherwise
13. Leave time for review

b. Essay questions
1. Read each question carefully
2. Determine exactly what is wanted. Underline key words or phrases.
3. Decide on outline or paragraph answer
4. Include many different points and elements unless asked to develop any one or two points or elements
5. Show impartiality by giving pros and cons unless directed to select one side only
6. Make and write down any assumptions you find necessary to answer the questions
7. Watch your English, grammar, punctuation and choice of words
8. Time your answers; don't crowd material

8) Answering the essay question

Most essay questions can be answered by framing the specific response around several key words or ideas. Here are a few such key words or ideas:

M's: manpower, materials, methods, money, management
P's: purpose, program, policy, plan, procedure, practice, problems, pitfalls, personnel, public relations

a. Six basic steps in handling problems:
1. Preliminary plan and background development
2. Collect information, data and facts
3. Analyze and interpret information, data and facts
4. Analyze and develop solutions as well as make recommendations
5. Prepare report and sell recommendations
6. Install recommendations and follow up effectiveness

b. Pitfalls to avoid
1. Taking things for granted – A statement of the situation does not necessarily imply that each of the elements is necessarily true; for example, a complaint may be invalid and biased so that all that can be taken for granted is that a complaint has been registered
2. Considering only one side of a situation – Wherever possible, indicate several alternatives and then point out the reasons you selected the best one
3. Failing to indicate follow up – Whenever your answer indicates action on your part, make certain that you will take proper follow-up action to see how successful your recommendations, procedures or actions turn out to be
4. Taking too long in answering any single question – Remember to time your answers properly

EXAMINATION SECTION

VOCABULARY

COMMENTARY

An integral, staple part of tests of academic aptitude and achievement and of general and mental ability is the vocabulary question, which appears in varied forms, the most common being the synonym-type, in which the subject word is followed by a group of four (4) or five (5) question-words (or phrases), and the candidate is asked to choose the word (or phrase) from this group that is closest in meaning to the subject word.

A lesser-used variation of this form is the context-type, in which the word to be defined ("subject word") appears within the framework of a sentence or phrase and is likewise followed by four (4) or five (5) question-words, from which the candidate is to choose the correct synonym or definition.

This vocabulary section is concerned only with the synonym-type.

The synonym-type of vocabulary question is usually attended by the following directions.

"Each question in this part consists of a word printed in capital letters followed by four (five) words lettered A, B, C, D, (E). Choose the letter of the word that is most nearly the SAME in meaning to the word in capital letters, and blacken the appropriate space on your answer sheet."

According to the directions, the candidate is to find a synonym in each group for the capitalized word. How does he proceed? Quickly scanning the group, he must decide which one of them is closest in meaning to the subject word. Then he is to mark the appropriate space on his answer sheet.

But to cope successfully and facilely with the vocabulary question requires intensive study and effort, culminating in vocabulary power, the ability to discern and comprehend the meanings of words, including their nuances.

There are two general ways of increasing or improving one's vocabulary — the so-called incidental method, whereby the candidate enlarges his vocabulary by wide reading, and the direct method — employed here — whereby the candidate goes about learning and overlearning the meanings of words through directed effort and absorption, just as he would endeavor to learn any other subject matter.

All the Tests in synonyms that follow are meant to accomplish the increase of vocabulary through direct learning activities. Undertake each of the tests, analyze your mistakes, then try to fixate the correct meanings and definitions of the various words.

SUGGESTIONS FOR ANSWERING THE VOCABULARY (SYNONYM-TYPE) QUESTION
1. Since this is a test whose validity rests upon its ability to measure your power to reason with words, please accept without reservation the reality that the synonym answer is at best an approximation and not, in most cases, a true synonym. It is up to you to choose the MOST NEARLY correct answer or BEST answer (of the choices offered). Do not anticipate finding literal or exact definitions used in these questions. This is how and where your ability to think, to reason, and to select will be shown.
2. Be alert concerning the part of speech of the subject word and the question items. In almost all cases, the correct answer should be of the same part of speech (e.g., an adjective) as the subject or question word (e.g., an adjective). This is a quick and easy test or method to eliminate some of the possibilities in the items. (Violations of this rule have proved to be exceptional.)

3. Be sure that you do not make the usual mistake of seizing upon an antonym, which you readily recognize in the question group, when a synonym is called for. This is a favorite device of the examiners — to throw in ready antonyms in order to test the alertness and perspicacity of the candidate. Thus, in the question:

AMBIGUOUS

   A. explicit   B. lucid   C. unintelligible   D. perspicuous
   E. unequivocal ,

the CORRECT answer is C. unintelligible; all the other four items are antonyms opposites).

4. The synonym, to be correct, must be in the same state, that is, active or passive, transitive or intransitive, as the subject word. This is really a continuation of the thought contained in 2 above. Thus, in the question:

PALLIATE

   A. mitigate   B. aggravate   C. extenuated   D. allure   E. castifate,

the CORRECT answer is A. mitigate, not C. extenuated, since the latter word, although an equally acceptable synonym, is in the past tense while the subject word is in the present tense.

5. Perhaps the most important counsel for vocabulary study and increase is the candidate's self-imposed discipline to learn the meaning of each and every word (item) in the question; i.e., not only the meaning of the subject word, with its correct answer, but — just as firmly — all the other words in the group. For example, in section 4 above, not only should the candidate know that *palliate* means A. *mitigate*, but he should, at the same time, check and overlearn the meanings of the other words in the group, namely, *aggravate, extenuated, allure,* and *castigate*.

6. Nor is this the end of the learner's unselfish obligation to himself. To accomplish a dynamic and abiding increase in his vocabulary power, he should not be content with carrying out section 5 above in its bare essentials. Not only should he know that *palliate* and *mitigate* are synonyms, but he should learn that there are several other equally good synoynms for these words, e.g., *abate, allay, assuage, appease, diminish, extenuate, gloss over, lessen, lighten, moderate, mollify, pacify, reduce, relieve, screen, soften, soothe, still, tranquillize.*

   And going one step beyond, he should acquire some of the various antonyms (opposites) for these synonyms, e.g., *aggravate, augment, embitter, enhance, foment, heighten, increase, intensify, magnify, make worse.*

   In this way, the effect of his study will be a chain reaction: he will be adding ten synonyms or antonyms for each key word he overlearns. And who can know whether these words might, in fact, just become the actual subject words or question words in the vocabulary part of the examination?

7. Do not readily accept the too-easy answer, particularly where the subject is almost matched by a look-alike in the question items; e.g., DECRY ... descry; DEPRECATE ... depreciate; DISCREET ...discrete; INGENIOUS ... ingenuous; LITERAL ...littoral; VENAL ... venial.

8. You should make time on this type of question. A strong and confident facility in vocabulary should enable you to recognize synonyms at once. Perhaps, it is an axiom to state that if you cannot handle this type of question quickly and efficiently, you will not do well on the test as a whole.

9. The best way to answer the synonym-type question is to scan the possible answers and to decide immediately upon the correct one. This presupposes strength and maturity of vocabulary. Only where the meaning of the word has little or no connotation for the candidate, should he attempt, by trial and error, to examine each possible answer in turn.
The method then is: scan and answer.

SAMPLE QUESTIONS AND EXPLANATIONS

Here is a vocabulary question that is estimated to be fairly easy:

I. *Harmony* means, most nearly,

    A. rhythm   B. pleasure   C. discord   D. tolerance   E. agreement

EXPLANATION OF SAMPLE QUESTION I

The answer is E. *agreement*, which means harmony between people, thoughts, and ideas. None of the other choices is so close to *harmony* in meaning.

Choice A, *rhythm*, like harmony, has something to do with music. But rhythm represents time, the pattern of light and heavy beats. That is not what harmony means.

Choice B, *pleasure*, may be brought about by harmony, but it is not harmony.

Choice C, *discord*, is the opposite of harmony.

Choice D, *tolerance* means getting along, but there is a difference between just barely getting along and being on the same beam as in harmony.

Here is a question estimated to be difficult for the general population, but that has been answered correctly by about half of a college sample.

II. *Salient means*, most nearly,

    A. prominent   B. vain   C. salty   D. liquid   E. clever

EXPLANATION OF SAMPLE QUESTION II

Choice A, *prominent*, like salient, means standing out, and is the correct answer.

Choice B, *vain*, may remind you of someone who is conceited, who thinks he stands out, but vain does not mean salient.

Choice C, *salty*, may remind one of saline which looks like salient but doesn't mean anything like it.

Choice D, *liquid*, also doesn't have any meaning in common with salient.

Choice E, *clever*, means showing deftness, skill, wit, or ingenuity -- not necessarily standing out.

III. *Circumvent* means, most nearly,

A. hasten	B. outwit	C. convince
D. accomplishment	E. outrun	

EXPLANATION OF SAMPLE QUESTION III

Choice A, *hasten*, and Choice C, *convince*, may be immediately discarded because of no relation to the question word.

Choice B, *outwit*, is the correct answer. The student with a background in Latin knows that the word *circumvent* is derived from *circum*, meaning *around*, and *venire*, *to come*, that is, *to come around*. This word has come to mean, in our language, *to frustrate*, that is, *to outwit*. Thus, we have discovered a synonym for *circumvent* in Choice B, *outwit*.

Choice D, *accomplishment*, should not be considered at all since it is not the same part of speech (it is a noun) as the question word (which is a verb).

Choice E, *outrun*, may present a momentary difficulty for decision because it contains a motion of movement somewhat similar to the basic meaning contained in the word *circumvent*.

IV. *Coeval* means, most nearly,

A. villainous	B. stealthy	C. contemporaneous
D. medieval	E. co-owner	

EXPLANATION OF SAMPLE QUESTION IV

Choice A, *villainous*, is meant to mislead because of the -eval in *coeval*.
Choice B, *stealthy*, is meant to mislead in the same way as Choice A.
Choice C, *contemporaneous*, is the correct answer.
Choice D, *medieval*, (from the Latin *medius*, middle, + *aevum*, age, "of or pertaining to the Middle Ages"), has merit but obviously is out of line so far as the time element is concerned.

V. *Clement* means, most nearly,

A. merciful   B. clemency   C. unreasonable   D. clamorous
E. acclimated

EXPLANATION OF SAMPLE QUESTION V

Choice A, *merciful*, is correct. *clement* (from the Latin *clemens*, mild, calm) means *merciful, lenient, mild (of weather)*. We immediately discern a synonym in Choice A.

Choice B, *clemency*, while it is the noun from which the adjective clement comes, must be discarded by the rules of the game since it is a different part of speech.

Choice C, *unreasonable*, has no valid connection with the subject word.

Choice D, *clamorous* (noisy, vociferous), is likewise to be disregarded.

Choice E, *acclimated* (to become used to a new environmental condition), has no connection save through some similarity in sound with the subject word.

VOCABULARY
EXAMINATION SECTION
TEST 1

DIRECTIONS: In each of the following word groups in this part, the word in each group is followed by four lettered words. In each group, select the lettered word that MOST NEARLY defines the capitalized word. *PRINT THE LETTER OF THE CORRECT ANSWER IN THE SPACE AT THE RIGHT.*

1. ACCOLADE
   A. jousting   B. soft drink   C. hubbub   D. praise   E. breach

   1._____

2. ACME
   A. grandiloquence   B. acne
   C. lowest point   D. prototype
   E. summit

   2._____

3. ALIMENTARY
   A. primary   B. mourning   C. charitable   D. nutritive   E. elementary

   3._____

4. ALTRUISM
   A. unselfishness   B. fanaticism
   C. honesty   D. inconstancy
   E. loyalty

   4._____

5. AMALGAM
   A. crime   B. rich mine   C. mixture   D. structure   E. cordon

   5._____

6. ANTIPATHY
   A. melancholy   B. musical response
   C. dislike   D. anger
   E. allurement

   6._____

7. BAROQUE
   A. grotesque   B. legalistic   C. dignified   D. plain   E. baronial

   7._____

8. BELLICOSE
   A. literary   B. pugnacious   C. comely   D. loud   E. bucolic

   8._____

9. BIGOTED
   A. intolerant   B. profane   C. corrupted   D. subdued   E. errant

   9._____

10. CAPTIOUS
    A. heroic   B. false
    C. authoritative   D. categoric
    E. hypercritical

    10._____

5

11. CORTEGE

    A. retinue
    B. artistic abstraction
    C. outer layer
    D. bouquet
    E. chameleon

12. CRYPTIC

    A. grave
    B. adverse
    C. germ destroying
    D. reticent
    E. occult

13. CUL-DE-SAC

    A. bottomless pit
    B. blind alley
    C. selective process
    D. old bag
    E. cult of personality

14. DECORUM

    A. basis of military award
    B. decorative scheme
    C. dogmatic order
    D. contrary to custom
    E. conformity to accepted standards

15. EBULLIENT

    A. burnished   B. exhilarated   C. destructive   D. verbose
    E. abusive

16. ENDEMIC

    A. native   B. unusual   C. fatal   D. diseased   E. erratic

17. ENIGMATIC

    A. spontaneous   B. negative   C. puzzling   D. oppressed
    E. merciless

18. ENSUE

    A. litigate   B. inveigle   C. follow   D. defeat   E. precede

19. EPHEMERAL

    A. spiritual   B. sensational   C. sparkling   D. worldly
    E. temporary

20. EXECRABLE

    A. wasteful   B. extremely painful   C. abominable
    D. digressing   E. desirable

21. EXIGENCY

    A. scantiness
    B. obvious presence
    C. plea for assistance
    D. urgent need
    E. exclusion

22. EXTANT
    - A. existing now
    - B. unpremeditated
    - C. spanning
    - D. without force
    - E. extinct

23. GARGOYLE
    - A. waterspout B. antiseptic C. ogre D. cherub E. chimera

24. GERMANE
    - A. appropriate B. elusive C. cruel D. contagious E. repulsive

25. GIBE
    - A. jest B. sneer C. present D. imitate E. mumble

26. HIATUS
    - A. expanse
    - B. cluster of stars
    - C. gap
    - D. rock texture
    - E. hindsight

27. ICONOCLAST
    - A. sculptor B. high priest C. radical D. atheist E. sybarite

28. IGNOMINIOUS
    - A. uninformed B. shameful C. luminous D. anonymous E. inveterate

29. IMMOLATE
    - A. vie with B. burn C. supplicate D. immure E. sacrifice

30. IMPORTUNE
    - A. imply B. imprecate C. solicit D. influence E. impress

31. IMPUNITY
    - A. without blame
    - B. immodest
    - C. pushed forward
    - D. without power
    - E. with ease

32. INTRACTABLE
    - A. not fertile B. intrepid C. undemocratic D. reversible E. stubborn

33. MARE'S NEST
    - A. hoax B. ambush C. manger D. high perch E. cache

34. MARTINET
    - A. novice
    - B. baton wielder
    - C. puppet
    - D. taskmaster
    - E. hostler

35. MENDACIOUS
    A. lying   B. humble   C. restoring   D. begging   E. preening

36. MISCREANT
    A. short prayer
    B. error in reading
    C. criminal
    D. hybrid
    E. misdemeanor

37. MODICUM
    A. good behavior
    B. current method
    C. pattern
    D. measure
    E. small portion

38. NEFARIOUS
    A. famous
    B. unmentionable
    C. conspicuous
    D. wicked
    E. furious

39. NOISOME
    A. offensive
    B. very loud
    C. inopportune
    D. argumentative
    E. exempt

40. NUANCE
    A. a shade of difference
    B. a simple dance
    C. the flounce of a skirt
    D. the height of fashion
    E. a new method

41. OVERT
    A. excited
    B. egg-shaped
    C. obverse
    D. opposite
    E. manifest

42. PECCADILLO
    A. tropical animal   B. slight offense   C. spicy relish
    D. embezzlement   E. prayer

43. PERFIDY
    A. completion   B. treachery   C. fragrance   D. indifference
    E. panoply

44. PERIPHERAL
    A. mysterious   B. half-tamed   C. external   D. wondering   E. perfidious

45. PRAGMATIC
    A. habitual
    B. flexible
    C. theological
    D. extemporaneous
    E. practical

46. PRODIGIOUS   46._____
    A. advantageous   B. wandering
    C. squandering   D. huge
    E. protean

47. PUNCTILIOUS   47._____
    A. scrupulous   B. prompt
    C. domineering   D. haughty
    E. picayune

48. PURVEY   48._____
    A. carry through   B. supply provisions   C. scrutinize
    D. encompass   E. purloin

49. RAMIFY   49._____
    A. render inviolate   B. arouse to anger
    C. reduce by means of heat   D. attack by collusion
    E. divide into branches

50. RESTIVE   50._____
    A. moving about   B. criticized   C. vacationing
    D. reconstructed   E. demanding

KEYS (CORRECT ANSWERS)

1. D	11. A	21. D	31. A	41. E
2. E	12. E	22. A	32. E	42. B
3. D	13. B	23. A	33. A	43. B
4. A	14. E	24. A	34. D	44. C
5. C	15. B	25. B	35. A	45. E
6. C	16. A	26. C	36. C	46. D
7. A	17. C	27. C	37. E	47. A
8. B	18. C	28. B	38. D	48. B
9. A	19. E	29. E	39. A	49. E
10. E	20. C	30. C	40. A	50. A

TEST 2

DIRECTIONS: In each of the following word groups in this part, the capitalized word in each group is followed by four lettered words. In each group, select the lettered word that MOST NEARLY defines the capitalized word. *PRINT THE LETTER OF THE CORRECT ANSWER IN THE SPACE AT THE RIGHT.*

1. PATINA
   - A. local guide
   - B. huckster
   - C. surface mellowing
   - D. dialect
   - E. pattern

2. PERMEATE
   - A. join an organization
   - B. conclude
   - C. take over leadership
   - D. spread through
   - E. design

3. PROLIFIC
   - A. profound
   - B. verbose
   - C. dissolute
   - D. original
   - E. fertile

4. PROSAIC
   - A. granting assent
   - B. of recent origin
   - C. metrical form
   - D. commonplace
   - E. prudent

5. PROSCENIUM
   - A. introduction to a tragedy
   - B. scenery for a play
   - C. forestage
   - D. satiric cartoon
   - E. prologue

6. PROVENDER
   - A. thrift
   - B. feed
   - C. offer
   - D. seller
   - E. buyer

7. ROSTER
   - A. list
   - B. voter
   - C. strutting leader
   - D. platform
   - E. bulwark

8. SALUTARY
   - A. seasoned
   - B. courteous
   - C. wholesome
   - D. oratorical
   - E. salivary

9. SAVOIR-FAIRE
   - A. aplomb
   - B. redemption
   - C. righteousness
   - D. animation
   - E. diffidence

10. SOLSTICE
    - A. furthest point
    - B. seclusion
    - C. healing mixture
    - D. seasonable weather
    - E. pertaining to the sun

11. SOPORIFIC
    - A. stimulating
    - B. narcotic
    - C. superficial
    - D. saturated
    - E. simplistic

12. STYPTIC
    A. germ destroying B. secret
    C. astringent D. putrid
    E. stifling

13. TERSE
    A. vivid B. unrelaxed C. compact D. prolix E. turgid

14. TORTUOUS
    A. rushing in a rapid stream B. very slow-moving
    C. dormant D. tenuous
    E. winding

15. UMBRAGE
    A. resentment B. artist's pigment C. nucleus of a sunspot
    D. obscurity E. cover

16. UNGAINLY
    A. ugly B. awkward C. long-legged D. underpaid
    E. unprofitable

17. VACILLATE
    A. interject B. prepare for occupancy C. lubricate
    D. brace E. waver

18. VIE
    A. blame B. question C. live D. contend E. violate

19. VOLATILE
    A. heavy B. wishful C. dangerous D. lively E. venomous

20. VORACIOUS
    A. shrewish B. truthful C. greedy D. eddying E. salacious

21. MADRIGAL
    A. song B. garland C. wine D. maiden E. carrousel

22. MERETRICIOUS
    A. easily influenced B. worthy
    C. uxorious D. victorious
    E. falsely alluring

23. MOLLIFY
    A. mutter B. appease C. tremble D. aggravate E. ruffle

24. NEOPHYTE
    A. new species B. beginner C. marine plant D. visitor
    E. blight

25. ONEROUS
    A. egotistic   B. commendable   C. burdensome   D. single
    E. meritorious

26. PALLIATE
    A. become very wan   B. rest comfortable   C. cure permanently
    D. parade ostentatiously   E. reduce in intensity

27. PERADVENTURE
    A. by accident   B. in danger   C. under oath
    D. through courage   E. with distinction

28. PEREGRINATE
    A. travel   B. penetrate   C. flounder   D. hibernate
    E. gravitate

29. PERSPICACIOUS
    A. optical   B. lucid
    C. spiny   D. keen
    E. conspicuous

30. POTABLE
    A. thick   B. edible
    C. drinkable   D. suited for cooking
    E. preliminary

31. PREDILECTION
    A. promise   B. weakness
    C. forecast   D. liking
    E. prescription

32. PURLOIN
    A. cleanse   B. steal   C. knit   D. stain   E. purvey

33. RANCOR
    A. rectitude   B. heart ailment
    C. acidity   D. unpleasant odor
    E. ill will

34. REGALE
    A. ennoble   B. upbraid   C. shout   D. enrage   E. entertain

35. SARDONIC
    A. descriptive   B. derisive   C. like a gem   D. fleshy
    E. gusty

36. SCRUPULOUS
    A. upright   B. exact   C. dishonest   D. neat and clean
    E. shrewish

37. SEMANTIC
    A. related to race   B. reproductive
    C. pertaining to meaning   D. uncivilized   E. ranting

38. SUPERCILIOUS
    A. rich   B. of the forehead   C. very stupid
    D. maculate   E. haughty

39. TAWDRY
    A. cheap and gaudy   B. worthless   C. obscene
    D. reddish brown   E. tepid

40. TRUCULENT
    A. ferocious   B. humble   C. immense   D. juicy   E. succulent

41. VICARIOUS
    A. vitreous   B. imaginary   C. neighborly   D. self-imposed
    E. substituted

42. VISCID
    A. smoky   B. sticky   C. internal   D. tainted   E. impetuous

43. VITIATE
    A. slander   B. impair   C. scratch   D. enliven   E. infuse

44. WHITE ELEPHANT
    A. valuable gift   B. troublesome possession
    C. retentive memory   D. faithful servant
    E. spotless reputation

45. WRAITH
    A. urchin   B. garment   C. valise   D. apparition   E. wick

46. UNEQUIVOCAL
    A. unpopular   B. indecisive   C. dubious   D. well-intentioned
    E. definite

47. VAGARIES
    A. wanderers   B. obscurities   C. fibers   D. caprices   E. whorls

48. VALANCE
    A. courage   B. degree of power
    C. worth   D. reward
    E. drapery

49. VIGNETTE
    A. spice or flavor   B. small house   C. hair dress
    D. small picture   E. tight housing

50. VITIATE
   A. produce acid
   B. corrupt
   C. enliven
   D. make unnecessary
   E. pervade

KEYS (CORRECT ANSWERS)

1. C	11. B	21. A	31. D	41. E
2. D	12. C	22. E	32. B	42. B
3. E	13. C	23. B	33. E	43. B
4. D	14. E	24. B	34. E	44. B
5. C	15. A	25. C	35. B	45. D
6. B	16. B	26. E	36. B	46. E
7. A	17. E	27. A	37. C	47. D
8. C	18. D	28. A	38. E	48. E
9. A	19. D	29. D	39. A	49. D
10. A	20. C	30. C	40. A	50. B

TEST 3

DIRECTIONS: In each of the following word groups in this part, the capitalized word in each group is followed by four lettered words. In each group, select the lettered word that MOST NEARLY defines the capitalized word. *PRINT THE LETTER OF THE CORRECT ANSWER IN THE SPACE AT THE RIGHT.*

1. ABJURE

    A. swear falsely
    B. charge solemnly
    C. absolve
    D. appeal
    E. renounce

    1._____

2. AERIE

    A. fantasy
    B. sprite
    C. purple flower
    D. eagle's nest
    E. hidden chamber

    2._____

3. AFFINITY

    A. preciseness   B. allergy   C. kinship   D. boundlessness
    E. affluence

    3._____

4. AMORPHOUS

    A. having no shape or form
    B. like powdered chalk
    C. sleep inducing
    D. rejecting another's caress
    E. colorless

    4._____

5. APATHY

    A. short, pithy statement   B. empathy   C. alertness
    D. non-symptom   E. indifference

    5._____

6. ARGOSY

    A. collection of tales
    B. watchful guardian
    C. bizarre adventure
    D. journey
    E. fleet of vessels

    6._____

7. ASCETIC

    A. characterized by acid taste
    B. occurring by chance
    C. self-denying
    D. rich in vitamins
    E. ministerial

    7._____

8. ASSIDUOUS

    A. bitter   B. obstinate   C. diligent   D. stupid   E. abstemious

    8._____

9. CAMBRIC

    A. mechanical device
    B. loose-fitting shirt
    C. two-wheeled vehicle
    D. cotton or linen fabric
    E. ancient custom

    9._____

10. CANTATA

    A. music drama   B. lead performer   C. popular card game
    D. female singer   E. salacious story

    10._____

15

2 (#3)

11. CHALICE
    A. decorative over-shirt B. small wooden cottage
    C. lightweight wool fabric D. drinking cup E. sacred emblem

12. CLAVICHORD
    A. harmonious arrangement B. term in mathematics
    C. early piano D. collar bone
    E. church indulgence

13. COGENT
    A. wistful B. ascertainable C. deceiving D. cognizant
    E. convincing

14. COLLUSION
    A. antagonism B. fraud C. mixture D. accident E. contumely

15. DECLAIM
    A. harangue B. disown C. greet D. challenge E. descry

16. DETERIORATE
    A. turn aside B. grow worse C. expand D. hold back
    E. aggrandize

17. DROLL
    A. provoking laughter B. misshapen creature C. expand
    D. hold back E. risque

18. EFFETE
    A. womanly B. exhausted C. festive D. mundane E. fetid

19. EFFUSIVE
    A. gushing B. vulgar C. revolutionary D. reserved
    E. glowing

20. ELICIT
    A. break the law B. plead for C. draw forth D. refine
    E. elide

21. ELISION
    A. apparition B. impact C. formation D. revision
    E. omission

22. EMPIRICAL
    A. authoritative B. scientific C. experiential D. maximal
    E. epistolary

23. EMPORIUM 23.____
    A. quack's office   B. altar canopy   C. absolute power
    D. commercial center   E. logical reasoning

24. ENERVATE 24.____
    A. weaken   B. insult   C. invigorate   D. introduce   E. impel

25. EXOTIC 25.____
    A. highly seasoned   B. amatory
    C. foreign   D. unbalanced
    E. eponymous

26. FACILITATE 26.____
    A. increase capacity   B. make safe   C. congratulate
    D. make easy   E. fructify

27. FALLACIOUS 27.____
    A. deadly   B. unwholesome   C. misleading
    D. deficient or lacking   E. factious

28. FLATULENT 28.____
    A. vapid   B. insipid   C. bombastic   D. limp   E. flocculent

29. FORTUITOUS 29.____
    A. lucky   B. couraeous   C. strong   D. accidental   E. finite

30. GREGARIOUS 30.____
    A. scanty   B. chanting rhythmically   C. flagrant
    D. corpulent   E. flocking together

31. HAPLESS 31.____
    A. incompetnt   B. unlucky   C. idiotic   D. careless
    E. haphazard

32. HARBINGER 32.____
    A. musket   B. street cleaner   C. bird   D. forerunner
    E. follower

33. ILLEGIBLE 33.____
    A. not literate   B. unqualified   C. undecipherable
    D. unacceptable   E. illicit

34. IMBROGLIO 34.____
    A. style of painting   B. seraglio   C. harem
    D. engraved gem   E. quarrel

35. IMPECCABLE 35.____
    A. irresistible   B. deficient   C. imperfect   D. faultless
    E. incomprehensible

36. INCUBUS
    A. evil spirit
    B. mathematical procedure
    C. hatching apparatus
    D. rain-bearing cloud
    E. bubonic plague

37. INEFFABLE
    A. inexpressible   B. uncouth   C. valueless   D. ruthless
    E. indefeasible

38. INGENUOUS
    A. without pretense   B. shrewd   C. cleverly inventive
    D. deceitful   E. indigenous

39. LANYARD
    A. area used for feeding cattle   B. short length of rope
    C. part of a system of gears   D. dress fabric
    E. nautical lamp

40. LECTERN
    A. oration   B. reading desk   C. textbook of law
    D. prayer reading   E. pulpit

41. LOQUACIOUS
    A. patient   B. alkative   C. disobedient
    D. logically consistent   E. sagacious

42. MARITAL
    A. warlike   B. official   C. female   D. nautical   E. connubial

43. MENDICANT
    A. traveling singer   B. one who presents a petition
    C. one who lies   D. beggar   E. miser

44. NOVICE
    A. beginner   B. short work of fiction   C. cloud formation
    D. doorpost   E. prelate

45. OBSEQUIOUS
    A. succeeding   B. unruly   C. latent   D. ceremonious
    E. subservient

46. OBSOLETE
    A. partially concealed   B. indecent   C. opposite the sun
    D. antiquated   E. apposite

47. OBVIATE
    A. make passable   B. render invisible   C. forestall
    D. make apparent   E. refer

48. OMINOUS
    A. providing for many things
    B. sinister
    C. leaving out
    D. all powerful
    E. ubiquitous

49. OSCILLATE
    A. fluctuate   B. kiss   C. confuse   D. yawn   E. delay

50. PALPABLE
    A. patent   B. fluttering   C. guilty   D. sponge-like
    E. possible

48.____
49.____
50.____

KEYS (CORRECT ANSWERS)

1. E	11. D	21. E	31. B	41. B
2. D	12. C	22. C	32. D	42. E
3. C	13. E	23. D	33. C	43. D
4. A	14. B	24. A	34. E	44. A
5. E	15. A	25. C	35. D	45. E
6. E	16. B	26. D	36. A	46. D
7. C	17. A	27. C	37. A	47. C
8. C	18. B	28. C	38. A	48. B
9. D	19. A	29. D	39. B	49. A
10. A	20. C	30. E	40. B	50. A

TEST 4

DIRECTIONS: In each of the following word groups in this part, the capitalized word in each group is followed by four lettered words. In each group, select the lettered word that MOST NEARLY defines the capitalized word. *PRINT THE LETTER OF THE CORRECT ANSWER IN THE SPACE AT THE RIGHT.*

1. LACONIC

    A. fearful   B. portentous   C. milky   D. severe   E. concise

2. LEES

    A. small heaps   B. small flags   C. dregs   D. meadows
    E. locusts

3. LEGUME

    A. envoy   B. vegetable   C. artificial channel
    D. token of honor   E. ravine

4. LOGISTICS

    A. military transportation and supply
    B. root word analysis
    C. philosophy stressing linguistic analysis of science
    D. pertaining to the velocity of projectiles
    E. forensic science

5. LUSTROUS

    A. passionate   B. glossy   C. vigorous   D. pallid   E. ghoulish

6. MIASMA

    A. disease of the eyes   B. mark of infamy
    C. respiratory ailment   D. bottomless pit
    E. poisonous exhalation

7. MINION

    A. servile dependent   B. lovable rascal   C. kitchen drudge
    D. quorum   E. novice

8. MONSOON

    A. flat-bottom boat   B. lunar phase   C. seasonal wind
    D. musical instrument   E. fainting spell

9. MOPPET

    A. female servant
    B. unwholesome mental condition
    C. utensil for storing household equipment
    D. very young girl
    E. small crater

1.__
2.__
3.__
4.__
5.__
6.__
7.__
8.__
9.__

10. MORTISE

    A. embalm B. embarrass C. join securely D. humiliate
    E. sequester

11. NAIAD

    A. lowest point B. water nymph C. Eastern potentate
    D. person who lacks guile E. local yoke

12. NECROMANCER

    A. teller of tales B. grave digger
    C. magician D. worshipper of ancestors
    E. embalmer

13. NETTLE

    A. thwart B. belittle C. cuddle D. err E. irritate

14. OLIGARCHY

    A. order of succession by power B. government by the few
    C. state of lawlessness D. benevolent despotism
    E. corrupt regime

15. PENATES

    A. household deities B. five-angled figures
    C. contrite persons D. winged creatures E. fire tools

16. PRECEDENT

    A. chief officer B. anticipation of evil
    C. established mode of procedure D. predilection
    E. preciosity

17. PROLIX

    A. abundantly productive B. tediously long talk
    C. introductory statement D. elongated along a diameter
    E. perfunctory statement

18. QUANDARY

    A. tradition B. quartile C. limitation D. excavation
    E. dilemma

19. ROOK

    A. crow B. young recruit C. strong-flavored cheese
    D. unit of land measure E. rock

20. SCURRILOUS

    A. industrious B. scampering C. obdurate
    D. grossly abusive E. indecently exposed

21. SEDULOUS

    A. seductive   B. disobedient   C. inactive   D. worldly
    E. persevering

22. SENTENTIOUS

    A. terse   B. unnatural   C. quarrelsome   D. showy
    E. presumptuous

23. SIROCCO

    A. fancy leather   B. North African dance   C. tropical fruit
    D. hot, dry wind   E. strident call

24. SKITTISH

    A. superficial   B. fretful
    C. untidy   D. easily frightened
    E. scintillating

25. SKULK

    A. slink   B. hunt   C. distort   D. pout   E. track

26. SOPHISTRY

    A. flattering action or speech   B. affectation of manner
    C. varied presentation   D. escessive admiration
    E. misleading argument

27. SQUEAMISH

    A. stubborn   B. overscrupulous   C. churlish   D. inert
    E. petulant

28. STENTORIAN

    A. sarcastic   B. loud   C. authoritative   D. pessimistic
    E. riparian

29. SUBVERT

    A. destroy   B. censure   C. ward off   D. turn downward
    E. subscribe

30. SUCCINCT

    A. pithy   B. juicy
    C. following in series   D. fortunate
    E. tangential

31. SURPLICE

    A. satiety   B. subsidiary
    C. conjecture   D. projection
    E. ecclesiastical vestment

32. SYCOPHANT

    A. fanatic   B. flatterer   C. voluptuary   D. special pleader
    E. tyrant

33. TEMERITY

    A. self-command   B. rashness   C. bashfulness   D. fanaticism
    E. timidity

34. THERAPEUTIC

    A. preventive   B. anesthetic   C. having healing qualities
    D. scientific   E. tendentious

35. THROTTLE

    A. crowd   B. overturn   C. palpitate   D. choke   E. stigmatize

36. TORQUE

    A. civil wrong   B. small-brimmed hat
    C. force causing rotation   D. apathy   E. club

37. TREPIDATION

    A. encroachment   B. timidity   C. breach of allegiance
    D. fear   E. mensuration

38. TRICOT

    A. three-cornered hat   B. emblem   C. trireme
    D. slang expression   E. knitted fabric

39. TURBID

    A. sluggish   B. distended   C. disturbed   D. muddy   E. torpid

40. USURP

    A. seize unlawfully   B. lend money   C. occupy
    D. make use of   E. suppress

41. VAGARY

    A. person lacking in means   B. inaccuracy
    C. prediction of things to come   D. wandering
    E. whim

42. VAPID

    A. transitory   B. savory   C. insipid   D. motionles
    E. mercurial

43. VERSATILE

    A. poetic   B. many-sided   C. reversed   D. proficient
    E. recusant

44. VICISSITUDE

    A. verification   B. proximity   C. likeness   D. vileness
    E. variation

45. VIRAGO

    A. dizziness   B. small bird   C. vestibule   D. country dance
    E. termagant

46. VIRTUOSO

    A. person of high morals   B. amateur
    C. orchestra leader   D. one skilled in the fine arts
    E. elder statesman

47. VISCOUS

    A. vitriolic   B. greedy
    C. malicious   D. made from synthetic materials
    E. glutinous

48. VORTEX

    A. focal point   B. highest point   C. outer layer
    D. whirlpool   E. cortex

49. WREAK

    A. inflict   B. ruin
    C. extract   D. smell unpleasant
    E. wreathe

50. ZEALOUS

    A. envious   B. enthusiastic   C. suspicious   D. brutish
    E. zany

KEYS (CORRECT ANSWERS)

1. E	11. B	21. E	31. E	41. E
2. C	12. C	22. A	32. B	42. C
3. B	13. E	23. D	33. B	43. B
4. A	14. B	24. D	34. C	44. E
5. B	15. A	25. A	35. D	45. E
6. E	16. C	26. E	36. C	46. D
7. A	17. B	27. B	37. D	47. E
8. C	18. E	28. B	38. E	48. D
9. D	19. A	29. A	39. D	49. A
10. C	20. D	30. A	40. A	50. B

VOCABULARY
EXAMINATION SECTION
TEST 1

DIRECTIONS: In each of the following word groups in this part, the capitalized word in each group is followed by four lettered words. In each group, select the lettered word that MOST NEARLY defines the capitalized word. *PRINT THE LETTER OF THE CORRECT ANSWER IN THE SPACE AT THE RIGHT.*

1. ALIGN
   - A. bring into line
   - B. carry out
   - C. happen by chance
   - D. join together

2. CONTRACTION
   - A. agreement
   - B. denial
   - C. presentation
   - D. shrinkage

3. INTERVAL
   - A. ending
   - B. mixing together of
   - C. space of time
   - D. weaken

4. LUBRICATE
   - A. bend back
   - B. make slippery
   - C. rub out
   - D. soften

5. OBSOLETE
   - A. broken-down
   - B. hard to find
   - C. high-priced
   - D. out of date

6. RETARD
   - A. delay
   - B. flatten
   - C. rest
   - D. tally

7. SUBLIMATE
   - A. cool
   - B. subdue
   - C. elevate
   - D. regulate

8. HYPOTHESIS
   - A. a supposition
   - B. relation
   - C. provision
   - D. proof

9. APPARITION
   - A. storm
   - B. noise
   - C. phantom
   - D. threat

10. MORDANT
    - A. caustic
    - B. depressed
    - C. dying
    - D. unwholesome

11. AFFILIATE
    - A. afford
    - B. respect
    - C. complicate
    - D. join

12. IMPROVISE
    - A. account for
    - B. show conclusively
    - C. invent offhand
    - D. slow down

13. PUNCTUAL
    - A. usual
    - B. hollow
    - C. infrequent
    - D. on time

14. BENEFICIAL
    - A. popular
    - B. forceful
    - C. helpful
    - D. necessary

15. RELY
    - A. depend
    - B. do again
    - C. use
    - D. wait for

16. SPURIOUS
    - A. discreet
    - B. just
    - C. counterfeit
    - D. apparent

17. DESULTORY
    - A. aimless
    - B. loathsome
    - C. stifling
    - D. uninterested

18. TRENCHANT
    - A. besieging
    - B. dissimilar
    - C. hidden
    - D. sharp

19. SUFFICIENT
    - A. steady
    - B. short
    - C. enough
    - D. higher

20. PROMPT
    - A. weight
    - B. quick
    - C. slow
    - D. advance

21. PENDING
    - A. awaiting
    - B. enclosing
    - C. leaning
    - D. piercing

22. VENDOR
    - A. customer
    - B. inspector
    - C. manager
    - D. seller

23. TRITE
    - A. brilliant
    - B. unusual
    - C. funny
    - D. commonplace

24. FESTIVE 24.____
    A. edible   B. joyous   C. proud   D. serene

25. TRANQUIL 25.____
    A. confused   B. medicinal   C. peaceful   D. temporary

26. SPASM 26.____
    A. splash   B. twitch   C. space   D. blow

27. HEMORRHAGE 27.____
    A. bleeding   B. ulcer
    C. hereditary disease   D. lack of blood

28. STEALTHY 28.____
    A. crazed   B. flowing   C. sly   D. wicked

29. COALESCE 29.____
    A. unite   B. reveal   C. abate   D. freeze

30. COERCION 30.____
    A. caution   B. intention
    C. disagreement D. compulsion

KEY (CORRECT ANSWERS)

1.	A	16.	C
2.	D	17.	A
3.	C	18.	D
4.	B	19.	C
5.	D	20.	B
6.	A	21.	A
7.	C	22.	D
8.	A	23.	D
9.	C	24.	B
10.	A	25.	C
11.	D	26.	B
12.	C	27.	A
13.	D	28.	C
14.	C	29.	A
15.	A	30.	D

TEST 2

DIRECTIONS: In each of the following word groups in this part, the capitalized word in each group is followed by four lettered words. In each group, select the lettered word that MOST NEARLY defines the capitalized word. *PRINT THE LETTER OF THE CORRECT ANSWER IN THE SPACE AT THE RIGHT.*

1. AUXILIARY
   - A. unofficial
   - B. available
   - C. temporary
   - D. aiding

    1.___

2. DELETE
   - A. explain
   - B. delay
   - C. erase
   - D. conceal

    2.___

3. REFUTE
   - A. receive
   - B. endorse
   - C. disprove
   - D. decline

    3.___

4. CANDID
   - A. correct
   - B. hasty
   - C. careful
   - D. frank

    4.___

5. INFRACTION
   - A. violation
   - B. investigation
   - C. punishment
   - D. part

    5.___

6. OBJECTIVE
   - A. method
   - B. goal
   - C. importance
   - D. fault

    6.___

7. CONCUR
   - A. agree
   - B. demand
   - C. control
   - D. create

    7.___

8. JUSTIFY
   - A. defend
   - B. understand
   - C. complete
   - D. request

    8.___

9. INFER
   - A. impress
   - B. conclude
   - C. intrude
   - D. decrease

    9.___

10. CONSTRUE
    - A. suggest
    - B. predict
    - C. interpret
    - D. urge

    10.___

11. TRIVIAL
    - A. unexpected
    - B. exact
    - C. unnecessary
    - D. petty

    11.___

12. OPTIONAL
    - A. useful
    - B. voluntary
    - C. valuable
    - D. obvious

    12.___

13. SUBSEQUENT
    A. following
    B. successful
    C. permanent
    D. simple

14. REVISE
    A. introduce
    B. explain
    C. begin
    D. change

15. CONCISE
    A. hidden
    B. complicated
    C. compact
    D. recent

16. PROSPECTIVE
    A. anticipated
    B. patient
    C. influential
    D. shrewd

17. STIMULATE
    A. regulate
    B. arouse
    C. imitate
    D. strengthen

18. EXPEDITE
    A. exceed
    B. expand
    C. solve
    D. hasten

19. RENOUNCE
    A. remind
    B. raise
    C. reject
    D. restore

20. SURMISE
    A. inform
    B. suppose
    C. convince
    D. pretend

21. FLUCTUATE
    A. vary
    B. divide
    C. improve
    D. irritate

22. PERTINENT
    A. attractive
    B. related
    C. practical
    D. lasting

23. CENSURE
    A. confess
    B. count
    C. confirm
    D. criticize

24. DIRGE
    A. unveiling
    B. cleansing
    C. lament
    D. billow

25. ENCUMBRANCE
    A. accommodation
    B. perversion
    C. valance
    D. hindrance

26. BRUSQUE
    A. long
    B. abrupt
    C. dangerous
    D. unpleasant

27. ERRONEOUS

    A. illegal   B. unkind   C. inaccurate   D. unknown

28. VELOCITY

    A. vertical   B. distance   C. depth   D. rate

29. PARADOX

    A. seemingly contradictory   B. perfect
    C. old-fashioned   D. a metaphor

30. PHENOMENON

    A. model   B. event   C. wish   D. performance

KEY (CORRECT ANSWERS)

1.	D	16.	A
2.	C	17.	B
3.	C	18.	D
4.	D	19.	C
5.	A	20.	B
6.	B	21.	A
7.	A	22.	B
8.	A	23.	D
9.	B	24.	C
10.	C	25.	D
11.	D	26.	B
12.	B	27.	C
13.	A	28.	D
14.	D	29.	A
15.	C	30.	B

TEST 3

DIRECTIONS: In each of the following word groups in this part, the capitalized word in each group is followed by four lettered words. In each group, select the lettered word that MOST NEARLY defines the capitalized word. *PRINT THE LETTER OF THE CORRECT ANSWER IN THE SPACE AT THE RIGHT.*

1. IGNOMINIOUS
   - A. dishonorable
   - B. ignorant
   - C. celebrated
   - D. unknown

   1.____

2. INTANGIBLE
   - A. indirect
   - B. numerous
   - C. impalpable
   - D. assiduous

   2.____

3. SUCCINCT
   - A. weak
   - B. concise
   - C. haughty
   - D. dangerous

   3.____

4. MALIGNANT
   - A. wasteful
   - B. virulent
   - C. discontented
   - D. happy

   4.____

5. INFAMOUS
   - A. unknown
   - B. noted
   - C. incompetent
   - D. notorious

   5.____

6. EFFECT
   - A. influence
   - B. obliterate
   - C. affect
   - D. appearance

   6.____

7. DEDUCE
   - A. deduct
   - B. conclude
   - C. detect
   - D. think

   7.____

8. PERTINENT
   - A. incessant
   - B. significant
   - C. saucy
   - D. impudent

   8.____

9. CONDONE
   - A. confirm
   - B. approve
   - C. forgive
   - D. offend

   9.____

10. INTREPID
    - A. fearless
    - B. uninterrupted
    - C. steady
    - D. inherent

    10.____

11. LUCRATIVE
    - A. wealthy
    - B. false
    - C. fortuitous
    - D. profitable

    11.____

31

12. PERFUNCTORY
    A. routine
    B. prompt
    C. accomplished
    D. dangerous

13. IMPECCABLE
    A. incapable
    B. flawless
    C. criminal
    D. incompetent

14. OSTRACIZE
    A. cajole
    B. flaunt
    C. harden
    D. exile

15. PUGNACIOUS
    A. specific
    B. frightened
    C. quarrelsome
    D. hearty

16. COALESCE
    A. dispel
    B. blend
    C. sweeten
    D. expedite

17. PEER
    A. equal
    B. arbitrator
    C. helper
    D. wharf

18. VINDICATE
    A. demonstrate
    B. clear
    C. conquer
    D. sway

19. GNARLED
    A. stooped
    B. aged
    C. smooth
    D. knotted

20. TACIT
    A. weak
    B. tactile
    C. silent
    D. written

21. PREVARICATION
    A. judgment
    B. evasion
    C. revision
    D. blasphemy

22. GARRULOUS
    A. talkative
    B. gaudy
    C. fearful
    D. persuasive

23. VESTIGE
    A. garment
    B. goddess
    C. view
    D. trace

24. ABJECT
    A. awesome
    B. miserable
    C. challenging
    D. opposing

25. OSTENSIBLE
    A. insecure
    B. variable
    C. professed
    D. ominous

26. REJUVENATED

   A. rested   B. rewarded   C. relieved   D. renewed

27. DISPARAGES

   A. disturbs   B. deceives   C. teases   D. degrades

28. SPECTRUM

   A. spirit
   C. a sound
   B. suspicious
   D. a range of color

29. IMPULSION

   A. turbulence
   C. driving force
   B. alternation
   D. embarkation

30. EMERGENCE

   A. emendatory
   C. coming forth
   B. disappearing
   D. wrenching

KEY (CORRECT ANSWERS)

1.	A	16.	B
2.	C	17.	A
3.	B	18.	B
4.	B	19.	D
5.	D	20.	C
6.	D	21.	B
7.	A	22.	A
8.	B	23.	D
9.	C	24.	B
10.	A	25.	C
11.	D	26.	D
12.	A	27.	D
13.	B	28.	D
14.	D	29.	C
15.	C	30.	C

TEST 4

DIRECTIONS: In each of the following word groups in this part, the capitalized word in each group is followed by four lettered words. In each group, select the lettered word that MOST NEARLY defines the capitalized word. *PRINT THE LETTER OF THE CORRECT ANSWER IN THE SPACE AT THE RIGHT.*

1. STOLID
   A. silent   B. morose   C. impassive   D. upright

2. RESOLUTE
   A. firm   B. honest
   C. independent   D. wise

3. REMONSTRATE
   A. contradict   B. urge
   C. reprimand   D. protest

4. DELETERIOUS
   A. imaginary   B. harmful   C. hateful   D. removal

5. CHARY
   A. careful   B. afraid
   C. ineffective   D. reckless

6. IMPORTUNE
   A. search   B. question   C. seize   D. beseech

7. CULMINATION
   A. end   B. accumulation
   C. climax   D. guilt

8. INSIDIOUS
   A. ingratiating   B. detestable
   C. insulting   D. treacherous

9. IMPLY
   A. conclude   B. permit   C. suggest   D. declare

10. MACHINATION
    A. pulverizing   B. plot
    C. thought   D. mechanization

11. SALUTARY
    A. beneficial   B. decisive
    C. salty   D. introductory

34

2 (#4)

12. DILATORY
    A. expanding	B. receding
    C. contradictory	D. delaying

    12.____

13. PEREMPTORY
    A. limited	B. interminable
    C. authoritative	D. disputed

    13.____

14. SPECIOUS
    A. deceptive	B. category
    C. controversial	D. disrespectful

    14.____

15. GERMANE
    A. vague	B. powerful	C. formative	D. relevant

    15.____

16. PSYCHOSOMATIC
    A. having an hypnotic influence
    B. experiential
    C. involving a mind-body relationship
    D. tending to induce sleep

    16.____

17. HYPOTHECATE
    A. assume
    B. establish a tentative theory
    C. imagine
    D. pledge for security

    17.____

18. SCHIZOID
    A. rare type	B. split personality
    C. symptom	D. syndrome

    18.____

19. PSYCHOSIS
    A. psychic experience	B. mental function
    C. mental disorder	D. test of mental ability

    19.____

20. VICARIOUS
    A. effective	B. substitute
    C. vicious	D. unworthy

    20.____

21. SIMULATE
    A. postulate	B. induce	C. feign	D. condone

    21.____

22. DICHOTOMOUS
    A. fastened together	B. transferred
    C. withheld	D. cut in two

    22.____

23. AMBIVALENCE

    A. attraction and repulsion
    B. gathering together
    C. careful consideration
    D. ability to walk

24. PSYCHOLOGICAL COMPLEX

    A. an intellectual perception
    B. a complicated theory of behavior
    C. an emotional pattern
    D. a fully completed action

25. INTROVERTED

    A. interrelated   B. interspersed
    C. conflicting   D. turned inwards

26. INHIBITED

    A. blocked   B. concealed   C. inherited   D. released

27. SUBLIMATION

    A. security   B. substitute experience
    C. emotional tone   D. inherent part

28. BENEVOLENCE

    A. good fortune   B. well-being
    C. inheritance   D. charitableness

29. BLITHE

    A. wicked   B. merry   C. sweet   D. pretty

30. JEOPARDIZE

    A. offend   B. destroy
    C. discourage   D. endanger

31. DISSENT

    A. detain   B. make an accusation
    C. disagree   D. call back

32. PASSIVE

    A. inactive   B. impartial   C. gloomy   D. former

33. CHRONIC

    A. painful   B. hopeless   C. complex   D. lingering

34. INCUR

    A. wait for   B. happen again
    C. bring upon oneself   D. prevent from happening

35. MANIFEST
    A. likely
    B. evident
    C. accidental
    D. convenient

36. DISSIPATE
    A. absorb
    B. disturb
    C. expect
    D. squander

37. INSIGHT
    A. mistake
    B. understanding
    C. confidence
    D. investigation

38. SURMOUNT
    A. overcome
    B. come down
    C. undermine
    D. go together

39. ASTUTE
    A. shrewd
    B. fair
    C. sensitive
    D. cruel

40. INHIBIT
    A. replace
    B. illustrate
    C. restrain
    D. include

41. PERENNIAL
    A. superficial
    B. lasting for years
    C. pleasing
    D. requiring little attention

42. CONSOLIDATE
    A. correct
    B. review
    C. control
    D. unite

43. ACCRUE
    A. accumulate
    B. report
    C. delay
    D. pay

44. DIFFUSE
    A. distinct
    B. spread out
    C. twisted
    D. clinging to

45. MOMENTOUS
    A. welltimed
    B. late in arriving
    C. important
    D. temporary

46. INNOCUOUS
    A. inadequate
    B. cautious
    C. harmless
    D. protected

47. PROLIFIC
    A. expressive
    B. prompt
    C. skillful
    D. productive

48. SUPPLANT

   A. take the place of
   C. settle finally
   B. give an advantage to
   D. support strongly

49. INFRINGE

   A. approach   B. insist   C. copy   D. trespass

50. CONDONE

   A. connect closely
   C. follow up
   B. pardon
   D. anticipate

KEY (CORRECT ANSWERS)

1. C	11. A	21. C	31. C	41. B
2. A	12. D	22. D	32. A	42. D
3. D	13. C	23. A	33. D	43. A
4. B	14. A	24. C	34. C	44. B
5. A	15. D	25. D	35. B	45. C
6. D	16. C	26. A	36. D	46. C
7. C	17. D	27. B	37. B	47. D
8. D	18. B	28. D	38. A	48. A
9. C	19. C	29. B	39. A	49. D
10. B	20. B	30. D	40. C	50. B

TEST 5

DIRECTIONS: In each of the following word groups in this part, the capitalized word in each group is followed by four lettered words. In each group, select the lettered word that MOST NEARLY defines the capitalized word. *PRINT THE LETTER OF THE CORRECT ANSWER IN THE SPACE AT THE RIGHT.*

1. APPRAISE
   A. inform   B. evaluate   C. increase   D. decrease

2. IMPARTIAL
   A. strange   B. funny   C. fair   D. bad

3. INCENTIVE
   A. cash   B. fire   C. messenger   D. motive

4. INSUBORDINATE
   A. confusing   B. disobedient
   C. important   D. smart

5. REVISION
   A. change   B. decision   C. dream   D. retreat

6. SEMIANNUALLY
   A. four times in a year   B. three times in a year
   C. twice in a year   D. every other year

7. UTILIZE
   A. break   B. cook   C. reduce   D. use

8. VAGUE
   A. new   B. sure   C. old   D. uncertain

9. CENTRIFUGAL
   A. moving away from a center
   B. moving toward a center
   C. having a center
   D. without a center

10. INDUCE
    A. cause   B. stop   C. name   D. signal

11. PERTINENT
    A. wise   B. stormy   C. relevant   D. understood

12. ENUMERATE
    A. free   B. count   C. postpone   D. obey

13. DEPLETE
    A. hide   B. order   C. purchase   D. empty

14. DIVERSE
    A. average   B. varied   C. faulty   D. hollow

15. MESH
    A. engage   B. skip   C. spin   D. use

16. DISMANTLE
    A. lock up
    C. look over
    B. forget about
    D. take apart

17. INCIDENTAL
    A. casual
    C. infrequent
    B. necessary
    D. needless

18. ELASTIC
    A. resilient   B. reserved   C. tranquil   D. sterile

19. ERRATIC
    A. opinionated
    C. irregular
    B. mistaken
    D. abusive

20. OBDURATE
    A. yielding
    C. persistent
    B. penitent
    D. indefatigable

21. FLAGRANT
    A. weakening
    C. scourge
    B. conspicuous
    D. emblem

22. SIMULATE
    A. arouse   B. instant   C. insinuate   D. imitate

23. OSTENTATIOUS
    A. substantial
    C. unpretentious
    B. apparent
    D. adaptable

24. LUCID
    A. unconfined
    C. unfortunate
    B. deprived
    D. hazy

25. OBSESS
    A. return
    C. lack
    B. afflict
    D. intermission

26. ELUCIDATE   26._____
   A. smooth   B. clarify   C. free   D. demonstrate

27. DEXTEROUS   27._____
   A. skillful   B. fast   C. patient   D. careful

28. EVOLUTION   28._____
   A. science   B. abatement
   C. evil   D. development

29. DUCTILE   29._____
   A. hard   B. liquid   C. rigid   D. flexible

30. PERIMETER   30._____
   A. spherical   B. diagonal   C. surface   D. boundary

KEY (CORRECT ANSWERS)

1.	B	16.	D
2.	C	17.	A
3.	D	18.	A
4.	B	19.	C
5.	A	20.	A
6.	C	21.	B
7.	D	22.	D
8.	D	23.	C
9.	A	24.	D
10.	A	25.	B
11.	C	26.	B
12.	B	27.	A
13.	D	28.	D
14.	B	29.	D
15.	A	30.	D

VOCABULARY
EXAMINATION SECTION
TEST 1

DIRECTIONS: In each of the following word groups in this part, the capitalized word in each group is followed by four lettered words. In each group, select the lettered word that MOST NEARLY defines the capitalized word. *PRINT THE LETTER OF THE CORRECT ANSWER IN THE SPACE AT THE RIGHT.*

1. PUNCTUAL

    A. usual
    B. hollow
    C. infrequent
    D. on time

    1.____

2. BENEFICIAL

    A. popular
    B. forceful
    C. helpful
    D. necessary

    2.____

3. TEMPORARY

    A. permanently
    B. for a limited time
    C. at the same time
    D. frecuently

    3.____

4. INQUIRE

    A. order
    B. agree
    C. ask
    D. discharge

    4.____

5. SUFFICIENT

    A. enough
    B. inadequate
    C. thorough
    D. capable

    5.____

6. AMBULATORY

    A. bedridden
    B. left-handed
    C. walking
    D. laboratory

    6.____

7. DILATE

    A. enlarge
    B. contract
    C. revise
    D. restrict

    7.____

8. NUTRITIOUS

    A. protective
    B. healthful
    C. fattening
    D. nourishing

    8.____

9. CONGENITAL

    A. with pleasure
    B. defective
    C. likeable
    D. existing from birth

    9.____

10. ISOLATION

    A. sanitation
    B. quarantine
    C. rudeness
    D. exposure

    10.____

11. DISTILLATE

    A. dilute
    B. absorption
    C. precipitate
    D. condensate

12. RHEOSTAT

    A. recur
    B. resistance
    C. an animal
    D. stationary

13. RENDEZVOUS

    A. parade
    B. neighborhood
    C. meeting place
    D. wander about

14. EMINENT

    A. noted   B. rich   C. rounded   D. nearby

15. CAUSTIC

    A. cheap   B. sweet   C. evil   D. sharp

16. BARTER

    A. annoy   B. trade   C. argue   D. cheat

17. APTITUDE

    A. friendliness
    B. talent
    C. conceit
    D. generosity

18. PROTRUDE

    A. project   B. defend   C. choke   D. boast

19. FORTITUDE

    A. disposition
    B. restlessness
    C. courage
    D. poverty

20. PRELUDE

    A. introduction
    B. meaning
    C. prayer
    D. secret

21. SECLUSION

    A. primitive
    B. influence
    C. imagination
    D. privacy

22. RECTIFY

    A. correct   B. construct   C. divide   D. scold

23. TRAVERSE

    A. rotate   B. compose   C. train   D. cross

24. ADAPT
    A. make suitable B. advise
    C. do away with D. propose

25. CAPACITY
    A. need B. willingness
    C. ability D. curiosity

26. EXEMPT
    A. defend B. excuse C. refuse D. expect

27. CONFORM
    A. conceal from view B. remember
    C. be in agreement D. complain

28. DILEMMA
    A. decision B. mistake
    C. violence D. predicament

29. OPPORTUNE
    A. temporary B. timely C. sudden D. recent

30. DEVIATE
    A. turn aside B. deny
    C. come to a halt D. disturb

31. COMPILE
    A. confuse B. support C. compare D. gather

32. MANIPULATE
    A. attempt B. add incorrectly
    C. handle D. investigate closely

33. POTENTIAL
    A. useful B. possible C. welcome D. rare

34. AUTHORIZE
    A. write B. permit C. request D. recommend

35. ASSESS
    A. set a value on B. belong
    C. think highly of D. increase

36. CONVENTIONAL
    A. democratic B. convenient
    C. modern D. customary

4 (#1)

37. DEPLETE

    A. replace   B. exhaust   C. review   D. withhold

38. INTERVENE

    A. sympathize with   B. differ
    C. ask for an opinion   D. interfere

39. HAZARDOUS

    A. dangerous   B. unusual   C. slow   D. difficult

40. SUBSTANTIATE

    A. replace   B. suggest   C. verify   D. suffer

41. DISCORD

    A. remainder   B. disagreement
    C. pressure   D. dishonest

42. TENACIOUS

    A. vicious   B. irritable
    C. truthful   D. unyielding

43. ALLEVIATE

    A. relieve   B. appreciate
    C. succeed   D. admit

44. FALLACY

    A. basis   B. false idea
    C. guilt   D. lack of respect

45. SCRUTINIZE

    A. reject   B. bring about
    C. examine   D. insist upon

46. IMMINENT

    A. anxious   B. well-known
    C. important   D. about to happen

47. SANCTION

    A. approval   B. delay   C. priority   D. veto

48. EGOTISTIC

    A. tiresome   B. self-centered
    C. sly   D. smartly attired

49. TRITE

    A. brilliant   B. unusual
    C. funny   D. commonplace

50. FESTIVE   50.____
    A. edible   B. joyous   C. proud   D. serene

KEY (CORRECT ANSWERS)

1. D	11. D	21. D	31. D	41. B
2. C	12. B	22. A	32. C	42. D
3. B	13. C	23. D	33. B	43. A
4. C	14. A	24. A	34. B	44. B
5. A	15. D	25. C	35. A	45. C
6. C	16. B	26. B	36. D	46. D
7. A	17. B	27. C	37. B	47. A
8. D	18. A	28. D	38. D	48. B
9. D	19. C	29. B	39. A	49. D
10. B	20. A	30. A	40. C	50. B

TEST 2

DIRECTIONS: In each of the following word groups in this part, the capitalized word in each group is followed by four lettered words. In each group, select the lettered word that MOST NEARLY defines the capitalized word. *PRINT THE LETTER OF THE CORRECT ANSWER IN THE SPACE AT THE RIGHT.*

1. SYNCHRONIZE

   A. draw out
   C. move at a steady rate
   B. happen at the same time
   D. turn smoothly

   1.___

2. OSCILLATE

   A. attract   B. echo   C. roll   D. swing

   2.___

3. TERMINAL

   A. last   B. moldy   C. named   D. spoken

   3.___

4. ADJACENT

   A. near   B. critical   C. sensitive   D. sharp

   4.___

5. AUTHORIZED

   A. false   B. permitted   C. powerful   D. written

   5.___

6. DETERIORATE

   A. decorate   B. prevent   C. regulate   D. worsen

   6.___

7. FLEXIBLE

   A. mixed
   C. not rigid
   B. not expensive
   D. solid

   7.___

8. NEGLIGENT

   A. careless   B. painful   C. pleasant   D. positive

   8.___

9. LOATHE

   A. rest   B. lend   C. hate   D. bother

   9.___

10. QUERULOUS

    A. complaining
    C. justified
    B. predictable
    D. oversized

    10.___

11. INHIBIT

    A. replace
    C. restrain
    B. illustrate
    D. include

    11.___

12. PERENNIAL

    A. superficial
    C. pleasing
    B. lasting for years
    D. requiring little attention

    12.___

13. CONSOLIDATE
    A. correct   B. review   C. control   D. unite

14. ACCRUE
    A. accumulate   B. report
    C. delay   D. pay

15. DIFFUSE
    A. distinct   B. spread out
    C. twisted   D. clinging to

16. MOMENTOUS
    A. welltimed   B. late in arriving
    C. important   D. temporary

17. INNOCUOUS
    A. inadequate   B. cautious
    C. harmless   D. protected

18. PROLIFIC
    A. expressive   B. prompt
    C. skillful   D. productive

19. SUPPLANT
    A. take the place of   B. give an advantage to
    C. settle finally   D. support strongly

20. INFRINGE
    A. approach   B. insist   C. copy   D. trespass

21. CONDONE
    A. connect closely   B. pardon
    C. follow up   D. anticipate

22. DISSENT
    A. detain   B. make an accusation
    C. disagree   D. call back

23. PASSIVE
    A. inactive   B. impartial   C. gloomy   D. former

24. CHRONIC
    A. painful   B. hopeless   C. complex   D. lingering

25. INCUR
    A. wait for   B. happen again
    C. bring upon oneself   D. prevent from happening

26. MANIFEST
    A. likely
    B. evident
    C. accidental
    D. convenient

27. DISSIPATE
    A. absorb
    B. disturb
    C. expect
    D. squander

28. INSIGHT
    A. mistake
    B. understanding
    C. confidence
    D. investigation

29. SURMOUNT
    A. overcome
    B. come down
    C. undermine
    D. go together

30. ASTUTE
    A. shrewd
    B. fair
    C. sensitive
    D. cruel

31. LOQUACIOUS
    A. grim
    B. talkative
    C. lighthearted
    D. hungry

32. PRECARIOUS
    A. violent
    B. uncertain
    C. troubled
    D. disastrous

33. SATURATE
    A. soak
    B. spoil
    C. filter
    D. dye

34. UNKEMPT
    A. untidy
    B. disagreeable
    C. uninformed
    D. crude

35. ORNATE
    A. enlightened
    B. watery
    C. decorated
    D. expensive

36. PANACEA
    A. stimulant
    B. disease
    C. remedy
    D. diagnosis

37. EQUITABLE
    A. equal
    B. just
    C. ordinary
    D. useful

38. DISTEND
    A. expand
    B. anger
    C. crush
    D. annoy

39. DERIDE
    A. remove
    B. jeer at
    C. cheer up
    D. hate

40. CRUX
    A. chief point
    B. strong action
    C. criticism
    D. desirable criterion

41. AVER
    A. consume   B. divert   C. defy   D. assert

42. APATHY
    A. sadness
    B. illness
    C. hunger
    D. indifference

43. ELATED
    A. lengthened
    B. matured
    C. excited
    D. youthful

44. SANCTION
    A. approval   B. delay   C. priority   D. veto

45. EGOTISTIC
    A. tiresome
    B. self-centered
    C. sly
    D. smartly attired

46. CAUTERIZE
    A. sear   B. melt   C. scrub   D. stoke

47. AVAILABLE
    A. lamentable
    B. traditional
    C. accessible
    D. fruitless

48. SUPPLEMENT
    A. terminal   B. absence   C. addition   D. void

49. HAZARDOUS
    A. dense   B. safe   C. dangerous   D. high

50. VERIFY
    A. climb   B. travel   C. slide   D. confirm

KEY (CORRECT ANSWERS)

1. B	11. C	21. B	31. B	41. D
2. D	12. B	22. C	32. B	42. D
3. A	13. D	23. A	33. A	43. C
4. A	14. A	24. D	34. A	44. A
5. B	15. B	25. C	35. C	45. B
6. D	16. C	26. B	36. C	46. A
7. C	17. C	27. D	37. B	47. C
8. A	18. D	28. B	38. A	48. C
9. C	19. A	29. A	39. B	49. C
10. A	20. D	30. A	40. A	50. D

TEST 3

DIRECTIONS: In each of the following word groups in this part, the capitalized word in each group is followed by four lettered words. In each group, select the lettered word that MOST NEARLY defines the capitalized word. *PRINT THE LETTER OF THE CORRECT ANSWER IN THE SPACE AT THE RIGHT.*

1. AMBIGUOUS
   A. separate B. uncertain C. improper D. lengthy

   1._____

2. INSTIGATE
   A. insult
   C. provoke
   B. find fault with
   D. examine closely

   2._____

3. RATIONAL
   A. sensible B. rapid C. meager D. impartial

   3._____

4. MITIGATED
   A. reinforced
   C. finished
   B. repaired
   D. softened

   4._____

5. INSULATE
   A. transfer B. insular C. isolate D. offend

   5._____

6. DUBIOUS
   A. doubtful
   C. duplicate
   B. uninterested
   D. ignorant

   6._____

7. ABRIDGE
   A. apply B. shorten C. adjust D. reach

   7._____

8. COMPRISE
   A. settle
   C. require
   B. be unaware of
   D. consist of

   8._____

9. INGRATIATE
   A. resent
   C. bring into favor
   B. show lack of appreciation
   D. lower

   9._____

10. TENACIOUS
    A. unyielding
    C. cruel
    B. anxious
    D. vague

    10._____

11. ALLEVIATE
    A. avoid B. relieve C. allow D. disagree

    11._____

12. ZEALOUS
    A. unselfish
    C. enthusiastic
    B. suspicious
    D. harsh

    12._____

13. DISSEMINATE
    A. copy B. discuss C. confirm D. spread

14. INNOVATE
    A. choose a plan of action B. introduce something new
    C. strengthen D. inspire

15. ASPIRATION
    A. solution B. recommendation
    C. preparation D. ambition

16. IMPLICATE
    A. impair B. agitate C. involve D. originate

17. SPURIOUS
    A. false B. serious C. inactive D. strange

18. EMULATE
    A. strive to equal B. arouse to action
    C. tear apart D. confide in

19. STRINGENT
    A. clear B. severe C. loose D. straight

20. VEHEMENT
    A. vidious B. honest C. calm D. intense

21. ELICIT
    A. act illegally B. draw forth
    C. expect D. erase

22. AUGMENT
    A. review B. arrange C. increase D. accept

23. PREVALENT
    A. rare B. unfair
    C. widespread D. correct

24. RECAPITULATION
    A. summary B. revision C. defense D. decision

25. ADVERSE
    A. unfavorable B. unwise
    C. anticipated D. backwards

26. COMMENDATORY
    A. expresses praise B. contains contradictions
    C. is too detailed D. is threatening

27. DEFER
    A. hasten B. consider C. postpone D. reject

28. MEAGER
    A. satisfactory B. scanty
    C. unexpected   D. praiseworthy

29. ARDUOUS
    A. requires much supervision
    B. is laborious
    C. absorbs one's interest
    D. is lengthy

30. IMPLICATED
    A. demoted B. condemned C. involved D. accused

31. DETAINED
    A. entertained B. held back
    C. sent away   D. scolded

32. AMIABLE
    A. active B. pleasing C. thrifty D. foolish

33. UNIQUE
    A. simple   B. uncommon
    C. useless D. ridiculous

34. REPLENISH
    A. give up B. punish C. refill D. empty

35. CONCISE
    A. logical B. favorable
    C. brief   D. intelligent

36. ELATED
    A. lengthened B. matured
    C. excited   D. youthful

37. ALLEGE
    A. raise B. convict C. declare D. chase

38. MENIAL
    A. pleasant B. unselfish C. humble D. stupid

39. DEPLETE
    A. exhaust B. gather C. repay D. close

40. ERADICATE
    A. construct B. advise C. destroy D. exclaim

41. CAPITULATE
    A. cover B. surrender C. receive D. execute

42. RESTRAIN
    A. restore B. drive C. review D. limit

43. AMALGAMATE
    A. join B. force C. correct D. clash

44. DEJECTED
    A. beaten B. speechless
    C. weak D. low-spirited

45. DETAIN
    A. hide B. accuse C. hold D. mislead

46. AMPLE
    A. necessary B. plentiful C. protected D. tasty

47. EXPEDITE
    A. sue B. omit C. hasten D. verify

48. FRAGMENT
    A. simple tool B. broken part
    C. basic outline D. weakness

49. ADVERSARY
    A. thief B. partner C. loser D. foe

50. ACHIEVE
    A. accomplish B. begin
    C. develop D. urge

KEY (CORRECT ANSWERS)

1. B	11. B	21. B	31. B	41. B
2. C	12. C	22. C	32. B	42. D
3. A	13. D	23. C	33. B	43. A
4. D	14. B	24. A	34. C	44. D
5. C	15. D	25. A	35. C	45. C
6. A	16. C	26. A	36. C	46. B
7. B	17. A	27. C	37. C	47. C
8. D	18. A	28. B	38. C	48. B
9. C	19. B	29. B	39. A	49. D
10. A	20. D	30. C	40. C	50. A

TEST 4

DIRECTIONS: In each of the following word groups in this part, the capitalized word in each group is followed by four lettered words. In each group, select the lettered word that MOST NEARLY defines the capitalized word. *PRINT THE LETTER OF THE CORRECT ANSWER IN THE SPACE AT THE RIGHT.*

1. FUNDAMENTAL 1.___
   A. adequate   B. essential   C. official   D. truthful

2. SUPPLANT 2.___
   A. approve   B. displace   C. satisfy   D. vary

3. OBLITERATE 3.___
   A. erase   B. demonstrate
   C. review   D. detect

4. ANTICIPATE 4.___
   A. foresee   B. approve   C. annul   D. conceal

5. EXORBITANT 5.___
   A. priceless   B. extensive   C. worthless   D. excessive

6. RELUCTANT 6.___
   A. anxious   B. constant   C. drastic   D. hesitant

7. PREVALENT 7.___
   A. current   B. permanent   C. durable   D. temporary

8. AUGMENT 8.___
   A. conclude   B. suggest   C. increase   D. unite

9. FRUGAL 9.___
   A. friendly   B. thoughtful
   C. hostile   D. economical

10. AUSTERITY 10.___
    A. priority   B. severity   C. anxiety   D. solitude

11. CORROBORATION 11.___
    A. expenditure   B. compilation
    C. confirmation   D. reduction

12. IMPERATIVE 12.___
    A. impending   B. impossible
    C. compulsory   D. logical

2 (#4)

13. FEASIBLE 13._____

   A. simple B. practicable
   C. visible D. lenient

14. SALUTARY 14._____

   A. popular B. urgent
   C. beneficial D. forceful

15. ACQUIESCE 15._____

   A. endeavor B. discharge C. agree D. inquire

16. DIFFIDENCE 16._____

   A. shyness B. distinction
   C. interval D. discordance

17. IDENTICAL 17._____

   A. named B. different
   C. exactly the same D. slightly bent

18. MAXIMUM 18._____

   A. most B. short C. proverb D. quiet

19. ANNUAL 19._____

   A. salary B. pension C. annoy D. yearly

20. INSPECT 20._____

   A. neglect B. vote C. examine D. possible

21. ADJACENT 21._____

   A. separate B. near
   C. look up to D. describe

22. EXCESSIVELY 22._____

   A. smaller than B. softer
   C. too much D. cool off

23. PARTIALLY 23._____

   A. friendly B. not completely
   C. soon D. exactly even

24. INDICATE 24._____

   A. cover up B. keep in C. increase D. point out

25. QUANTITY 25._____

   A. put out B. amount C. question D. excellent

59

26. VICINITY
    A. victory   B. far away
    C. examination   D. neighborhood

27. COMPEL
    A. return   B. accept   C. release   D. force

28. ACCURATE
    A. correct   B. measure   C. add up   D. easy

29. INSTANTLY
    A. too slowly   B. correctly
    C. right away   D. noisily

30. COOPERATE
    A. work together   B. prevent
    C. vote against   D. step back

31. INQUIRE
    A. ask   B. put off   C. insist   D. pass over

32. EXCESS
    A. dig   B. extra   C. fill   D. excuse

33. CONTRACT
    A. shrink   B. remove   C. enlarge   D. inspect

34. ROTATE
    A. control   B. return   C. protect   D. turn

35. REPLACE
    A. change   B. put back   C. open up   D. answer

36. SELECT
    A. repair   B. leave   C. choose   D. avoid

37. ATTEMPT
    A. connect   B. agree   C. support   D. try

38. DISPUTE
    A. argue   B. blame   C. lend   D. settle

39. DISTINCT
    A. clear   B. mixed   C. far away   D. difficult

40. FREQUENTLY
    A. unusual   B. late   C. friendly   D. often

41. INDICATE
    - A. hide
    - B. light
    - C. show
    - D. follow

42. REGRESS
    - A. retreat
    - B. deviate
    - C. intrude
    - D. transgress

43. TERMINOLOGY
    - A. termination
    - B. composition
    - C. nomenclature
    - D. punctuation

44. CATALOG
    - A. to list
    - B. to rate
    - C. to print
    - D. to price

45. DURABLE
    - A. smooth
    - B. sticky
    - C. lasting
    - D. feeling

46. MUTUAL
    - A. silent
    - B. shared
    - C. changing
    - D. broken

47. REJECT
    - A. rewrite
    - B. refuse
    - C. release
    - D. regret

48. OBSTRUCT
    - A. teach
    - B. darken
    - C. block
    - D. resist

49. CORRODE
    - A. melt
    - B. rust
    - C. burn
    - D. warp

50. EXCESS
    - A. surplus
    - B. storage
    - C. spacing
    - D. survey

KEY (CORRECT ANSWERS)

1. B	11. C	21. B	31. A	41. C
2. B	12. C	22. C	32. B	42. A
3. A	13. B	23. B	33. A	43. C
4. A	14. C	24. D	34. D	44. A
5. D	15. C	25. B	35. B	45. C
6. D	16. A	26. D	36. C	46. B
7. A	17. C	27. D	37. D	47. B
8. C	18. A	28. A	38. A	48. C
9. D	19. D	29. C	39. A	49. B
10. B	20. C	30. A	40. D	50. A

TEST 5

DIRECTIONS: In each of the following word groups in this part, the capitalized word in each group is followed by four lettered words. In each group, select the lettered word that MOST NEARLY defines the capitalized word. *PRINT THE LETTER OF THE CORRECT ANSWER IN THE SPACE AT THE RIGHT.*

1. VARIATION
    A. change
    B. representative
    C. simplification
    D. trial

    1.____

2. CREDIBLE
    A. believable
    B. impossible
    C. payable
    D. understandable

    2.____

3. SUBTERFUGE
    A. argument   B. deception   C. excuse   D. flight

    3.____

4. CONCISE
    A. brief   B. mixed   C. sarcastic   D. split

    4.____

5. SPURIOUS
    A. angry   B. evident   C. false   D. odd

    5.____

6. INCOHERENT
    A. damaged
    B. fearful
    C. inside
    D. uncoordinated

    6.____

7. CORROBORATE
    A. confirm   B. confuse   C. decay   D. defraud

    7.____

8. GRATUITY
    A. favor   B. greeting   C. scheme   D. tip

    8.____

9. ALTERCATION
    A. angry dispute
    B. recent change
    C. renewal
    D. substitution

    9.____

10. ASCERTAIN
    A. authorize   B. determine   C. provide   D. publish

    10.____

11. DISCRIMINATE
    A. involve in crime
    B. spread widely
    C. test repeatedly
    D. treat differently

    11.____

12. DIVULGE
    A. reveal   B. separate   C. share   D. swell

    12.____

13. EMBARGO
    A. container B. license C. load D. stoppage

14. CENSURE
    A. anxiety B. blame C. middle D. pause

15. CALIBRATE
    A. check someone else's calculations
    B. derive a formula to give desired results
    C. make calculations after inaccurate measurements have been taken
    D. mark appropriate graduations on a measuring instrument

16. EJECT
    A. contest B. refuse C. give in D. throw out

17. MERCANTILE
    A. advertising B. commercial
    C. discount D. wholesale

18. REQUISITION
    A. deny B. recognition
    C. request D. surrender

19. PROMULGATE
    A. agree to B. publish C. spend D. veto

20. EXCLUDE
    A. go over B. keep out C. look up D. look out

21. RESUME
    A. begin again B. stop off
    C. take off D. take out

22. DISBURSEMENT
    A. quotation B. commission
    C. expenditure D. worsening

23. INVENTORY
    A. bill of sale B. itemized list
    C. delivery D. promotion

24. SUBSTANTIATE
    A. challenge B. take away C. prove D. increase

25. RESCIND
    A. approve B. cancel
    C. take part in D. remake

26. CONSOLIDATE

    A. divide in half   B. direct
    C. agree   D. unite

27. EXPEDITE

    A. label carefully   B. process promptly
    C. represent   D. terminate

28. GARRULOUS

    A. excited   B. questioning
    C. silly   D. talkative

29. ADMONISH

    A. remember   B. silence   C. urge   D. warn

30. OSTENSIBLE

    A. avowed   B. chief   C. extended   D. real

31. PRECARIOUS

    A. careless   B. thin
    C. uncertain   D. undesirable

32. INDIGENT

    A. destitute   B. disreputable
    C. lazy   D. stingy

33. ACRIMONIOUS

    A. bitter   B. loud
    C. rich   D. unjustified

34. INFER

    A. assume   B. conclude   C. indicate   D. state

35. FORTUITOUS

    A. accidental   B. desirable
    C. fortunate   D. strong

36. LUGUBRIOUS

    A. middle-aged   B. mournful
    C. ridiculous   D. sarcastic

37. PONDEROUS

    A. critical   B. effortless
    C. heavy   D. solid

38. PLENARY

    A. authoritative   B. executive
    C. full   D. important

39. LACONIC 39.____

    A. deliberate B. inattentive
    C. short   D. wise

40. INVIDIOUS 40.____

    A. deceptive B. offensive
    C. poor   D. serious

41. RAMBLE 41.____

    A. run   B. ride   C. crawl   D. roam

42. STERILE 42.____

    A. productive   B. stereotype
    C. feebleminded D. barren

43. ABOLISH 43.____

    A. count up   B. do away with
    C. give more   D. pay double for

44. ABUSE 44.____

    A. accept   B. mistreat   C. respect   D. touch

45. ACCURATE 45.____

    A. correct   B. lost   C. neat   D. secret

46. ASSISTANCE 46.____

    A. attendance B. belief
    C. help   D. reward

47. CAUTIOUS 47.____

    A. brave   B. careful   C. greedy   D. hopeful

48. COURTEOUS 48.____

    A. better   B. easy   C. polite   D. religious

49. CRITICIZE 49.____

    A. admit   B. blame   C. check on   D. make dirty

50. FLEXIBLE 50.____

    A. neatly folded B. easily broken
    C. easily bent   D. neatly piled

KEY (CORRECT ANSWERS)

1. A	11. D	21. A	31. C	41. D
2. A	12. A	22. C	32. A	42. D
3. B	13. D	23. B	33. A	43. B
4. A	14. B	24. C	34. B	44. B
5. C	15. D	25. B	35. A	45. A
6. D	16. D	26. D	36. B	46. C
7. A	17. B	27. B	37. C	47. B
8. D	18. C	28. D	38. C	48. C
9. A	19. B	29. D	39. C	49. B
10. B	20. B	30. A	40. B	50. C

ANTONYMS/OPPOSITES

COMMENTARY

The opposite-type question is one step further removed in difficulty from the synonym-type. Its greater difficulty is readily discernible when one considers that in order to answer as to the opposite, one must first know what the word means — that is, the synonym. Thus, a transitional stage in the thought process (the same) is skipped over, and one is compelled forthwith to move on to the next stage (the opposite) in the same amount of time allotted.

For this type of vocabulary question, it is not sufficient for the candidate to have merely a general knowledge of the meanings of words. It will be necessary for him to know their meanings with power and discrimination.

In the questions presented, the items or choices will be very closely related so that only a sure and precise understanding will lead to the correct answer. To the uninitiated, i.e., the candidate with average word-power, any one of the choices presented in the question will seem acceptable and each, in turn, will present individual difficulty, leading to uncertainty, confusion, and loss of time on a test for which definite time limits are assigned. Therefore, it is most important that the candidate reinforce his accustomed incidental learning of the meanings of words by directed, purposeful study and overlearning of vocabulary.

The opposite type of question is usually attended by the following directions:

DIRECTIONS: Each question in this part consists of a word in capital letters, followed by five words numbered 1 through 5. Choose the number of the word that is most nearly OPPOSITE in meaning to the word in capital letters, and mark the appropriate space on your answer sheet.

SUGGESTIONS FOR ANSWERING THE OPPOSITE (ANTONYM)-TYPE QUESTION

1. Since this is an aptitude test, whose validity rests upon its ability to measure your power to reason with words, please accept without reservation the reality that the antonym answer is at best an approximation and not, in most cases, a true opposite. It is up to you to choose the MOST NEARLY correct answer or BEST answer (of the choices offered). Do not anticipate finding literal or exact opposite meanings used in these questions. This is how and where your ability to think, to reason, and to select will be shown.

2. Be alert concerning the part of speech of the subject word and question items. In all cases, the correct answer should be of the same part of speech (e.g., an adjective) as the subject or question word (e.g., an adjective). This is a quick and easy test or method to eliminate some of the given possibilities in the question. (Violations of this rule in previous examinations have proved to be exceptional.)

3. Beware of choosing as an opposite a word which is broader or more limited in scope than the subject word. For example, in the question below:
  ECONOMICAL   1. deistic 2. liberal 3. lavish 4. frugal
                5. amicable,
the correct answer is 3. lavish, not 2. liberal. The reason for this is that while liberal is opposed to economical, it is too moderate in scope, denoting a quality not so adequately described as by

the word, lavish, which is on the extreme opposite end of the word-pole in relation to the subject word, economical.

4. The opposite, to be correct, must be in the same state, that is, active or passive, transitive or intransitive, as the subject word. This is really a continuation of the thought contained in (3) above. Thus, in the question:

ENTICE 1. detract 2. repelled 3. decoy 4. repulse 5. negate, the correct answer is 4. repulse, not 2. repelled, since the latter word is in the past tense, while the subject word is in the present tense.

5. Should the question call for an opposite, be sure that you do not make the usual mistake of seizing upon a synonym which you readily recognize in the question group, when an antonym is called for. This is a favorite device of the examiners to throw in ready synonyms in order to test the alertness and perspicacity of the candidate.

6. You should make time on this type of question. A strong and confident facility in vocabulary should enable you to recognize synonyms at once; antonyms should cause you to think, but, nevertheless, should take just a little longer than the synonym question. Perhaps, it is an axiom to state that if you cannot handle this type of question quickly and efficiently, you will not do well on the aptitude test as a whole.

7. The best way to answer the opposite type of question is to scan the possible answers and to decide immediately upon the correct one. This presupposes strength and maturity of vocabulary. Only where the meaning of the word has little or no connotation for the candidate should he attempt, by trial and error, to examine each possible answer in turn.

The formula then is: scan and answer.

ANTONYMS/OPPOSITES
EXAMINATION SECTION
TEST 1

DIRECTIONS: Each question below consists of a word printed in capital letters, followed by five words or phrases lettered A through E. Choose the lettered word or phrase that is *most nearly* OPPOSITE in meaning to the word in capital letters. *PRINT THE LETTER OF THE CORRECT ANSWER IN THE SPACE AT THE RIGHT.*

1. ACRID
    - A. smoky
    - B. withered
    - C. sharp
    - D. mild
    - E. acerb

   1.____

2. ALLERGY
    - A. extreme sensitivity
    - B. distaste
    - C. sleepiness
    - D. suppressed desire
    - E. unsusceptibility

   2.____

3. AMBIGUOUS
    - A. acoustic
    - B. ambivalent
    - C. equivocal
    - D. imitating
    - E. succinct

   3.____

4. AMELIORATE
    - A. bring together
    - B. settle a dispute
    - C. worsen
    - D. improve
    - E. amend

   4.____

5. AUGMENT
    - A. sever
    - B. disperse
    - C. increase
    - D. diminish
    - E. argue

   5.____

6. BANAL
    - A. sarcastic
    - B. trite
    - C. novel
    - D. futuristic
    - E. sagacious

   6.____

7. BEATIFY
    - A. make lovely
    - B. desecrate
    - C. make happy
    - D. restore
    - E. hallow

   7.____

8. BOURGEOIS
    - A. middle-class citizen
    - B. capital letters
    - C. swollen streams
    - D. nobility
    - E. peasant

   8.____

9. BROMIDE
    - A. vegetable
    - B. petty bribe
    - C. pamphlet
    - D. skin abrasion
    - E. epigram

   9.____

69

10. BRING

    A. fetch   B. transfer   C. relate
    D. suggest   E. dispatch

11. CAPRICIOUS

    A. fickle   B. fault-finding   C. sneering
    D. dominating   E. resolve

12. CASUAL

    A. watery   B. fated   C. fortuitous
    D. aromatic   E. moving

13. CHOLERIC

    A. dignified   B. high-tempered   C. gloomy
    D. unexcitable E. caustic

14. CIRCULAR

    A. muscular   B. oblique   C. grouped
    D. pivotal   E. incongruous

15. CIRCUMVENT

    A. succor   B. reserve   C. fortify
    D. surround   E. delude

16. COMPASSIONATE

    A. pitiful   B. merciful   C. ruthless
    D. reluctant   E. pietistic

17. COMPLIANCE

    A. violation   B. regulation   C. attendance
    D. submission   E. conformance

18. CONDIGN

    A. punishable   B. scheming   C. undeserved
    D. merited   E. condemn

19. CONDONE

    A. demand payment   B. express sympathy   C. forget
    D. revenge   E. forgive

20. COPE

    A. fail in striving   B. contend on equal terms
    C. plug with soft material   D. crown with laurel
    E. compare with others

21. DECOROUS

    A. unseemly   B. proper   C. low cut
    D. in groups of ten E. deteriorating

22. DESPONDENT
    A. powdery   B. bent   C. optional
    D. artificial   E. elated

23. DESULTORY
    A. pompous   B. methodical   C. rambling
    D. oppressively hot E. cursory

24. DETONATE
    A. explode   B. deafen   C. muffle
    D. fizzle out   E. destroy

25. DISCIPLE
    A. impostor   B. follower   C. antagonist
    D. paragon   E. colleague

KEYS (CORRECT ANSWERS)

1. D
2. E
3. E
4. C
5. D

6. C
7. B
8. E
9. E
10. E

11. E
12. B
13. D
14. B
15. A

16. C
17. A
18. C
19. D
20. A

21. A
22. E
23. B
24. C
25. C

TEST 2

DIRECTIONS: Each question below consists of a word printed in capital letters, followed by five words or phrases lettered A through E. Choose the lettered word or phrase that is *most nearly* OPPOSITE in meaning to the word in capital letters. *PRINT THE LETTER OF THE CORRECT ANSWER IN THE SPACE AT THE RIGHT.*

1. DISCREET
   - A. cautious
   - B. chary
   - C. prudent
   - D. distinct
   - E. temerarious

   1.___

2. DISINTER
   - A. dig up from a grave
   - B. lack interest
   - C. interrupt
   - D. inject between muscles
   - E. entomb

   2.___

3. DOGGEREL
   - A. trivial verse
   - B. small canine species
   - C. stubborn behavior
   - D. sophisticated poetry
   - E. manger

   3.___

4. DOLE OUT
   - A. squander
   - B. distribute piecemeal
   - C. control
   - D. deny alms
   - E. hoard

   4.___

5. DOMINEERING
   - A. dictatorial
   - B. pliant
   - C. considerate
   - D. unsympathetic
   - E. recreant

   5.___

6. ELEGY
   - A. inheritance
   - B. burnt offering
   - C. violin obbligato
   - D. dirge
   - E. paean

   6.___

7. ELICIT
   - A. concoct with alcohol
   - B. draw out
   - C. compel approval
   - D. request sharply
   - E. ignite

   7.___

8. EMOLLIENT
   - A. salve
   - B. monument
   - C. tariff charge
   - D. extra tip
   - E. abrasive

   8.___

9. ENCORE
   - A. intermission
   - B. termination
   - C. heart of the matter
   - D. repetition
   - E. variation

   9.___

10. ENERVATE
    - A. stumble
    - B. devitalize
    - C. stimulate
    - D. rejoice
    - E. impede

    10.___

11. EXPIATION   11.____
    A. reprobation   B. clarification   C. failure
    D. atonement   E. interpretation

12. FABULOUS   12.____
    A. wealthy   B. impressionistic C. realistic
    D. legendary   E. fictional

13. FAIRWAY   13.____
    A. airplane landing field   B. golf greensward   C. captain's private quarters
    D. entrance to ferry slip   E. coppice

14. FEASIBLE   14.____
    A. garish   B. festive   C. theoretical
    D. practicable   E. pertinent

15. FIERY   15.____
    A. vehement   B. irritable   C. restive
    D. gay   E. indifferent

16. FLORID   16.____
    A. flowing   B. livid   C. blotchy
    D. ruddy   E. over-heated

17. FLOUT   17.____
    A. move   B. mock   C. obey
    D. defy   E. flog

18. FOREGO   18.____
    A. prosecute   B. align   C. renounce
    D. look forward   E. over-heated

19. FURTIVE   19.____
    A. fleeing   B. hairy   C. glancing
    D. stealthy   E. ingenuous

20. GARBLE   20.____
    A. substantiate   B. garnish   C. mutilate
    D. unravel   E. embroider

21. GARRULOUS   21.____
    A. talkative   B. quarrelsome   C. snarling
    D. laconic   E. ungainly

22. GOSSAMER   22.____
    A. sleezy   B. dusty   C. gauzy
    D. unbreakable   E. zephyr-like

23. GOURMAND

    A. greedy eater   B. epicure   C. hungry person
    D. ascetic   E. fried pumpkin shell

23.____

24. GRIEVOUS

    A. rutty   B. gratifying   C. sorrowful
    D. vicious   E. unmentionable

24.____

25. GRIMACE

    A. happy smile   B. fruit sherbet   C. twisting of the countenance
    D. fine quality silk   E. sneer

25.____

KEYS (CORRECT ANSWERS)

1.	E	11.	A
2.	E	12.	C
3.	D	13.	E
4.	A	14.	C
5.	B	15.	E
6.	E	16.	B
7.	D	17.	C
8.	E	18.	A
9.	B	19.	E
10.	C	20.	A

21. D
22. D
23. D
24. B
25. A

TEST 3

DIRECTIONS: Each question below consists of a word printed in capital letters, followed by five words or phrases lettered A through E. Choose the lettered word or phrase that is *most nearly* OPPOSITE in meaning to the word in capital letters. *PRINT THE LETTER OF THE CORRECT ANSWER IN THE SPACE AT THE RIGHT.*

1. HEINOUS
    - A. criminal
    - B. elevated
    - C. inhuman
    - D. flagrant
    - E. moderate

    1._____

2. HUE
    - A. tint
    - B. shade
    - C. tone
    - D. tinge
    - E. etiolation

    2._____

3. IMMUNITY
    - A. protection against accident
    - B. exemption
    - C. freedom from disease
    - D. dispensation
    - E. tendency

    3._____

4. IMPLICIT
    - A. directly stated
    - B. understood though not expressed
    - C. omitted entirely by chance
    - D. stated but not for publication
    - E. inherent

    4._____

5. IMPUTE
    - A. insult
    - B. contradict
    - C. ascribe
    - D. question
    - E. refer

    5._____

6. INCIPIENT
    - A. tasteless
    - B. criminal
    - C. beginning
    - D. diseased
    - E. terminal

    6._____

7. INGENUOUS
    - A. guileful
    - B. naive
    - C. frank
    - D. uncertain
    - E. jealous

    7._____

8. INIQUITOUS
    - A. awesome
    - B. unequal
    - C. wicked
    - D. present everywhere
    - E. exemplary

    8._____

9. INTERMITTENT
    - A. continuing without break
    - B. occurring at intervals
    - C. persistently noisy
    - D. gradually subdued
    - E. intermediate

    9._____

2 (#3)

10. INTRANSIGENT 10.___
    - A. utterly fearless
    - B. irreconcilable
    - C. invalid
    - D. not transferable
    - E. tractable

11. INTREPID 11.___
    - A. fearful
    - B. uneasy
    - C. dauntless
    - D. stumbling
    - E. insistent

12. INURE 12.___
    - A. maim
    - B. entice
    - C. deplete
    - D. toughen
    - E. endure

13. INVOKE 13.___
    - A. provoke
    - B. denounce
    - C. slanderous
    - D. address in prayer
    - E. evoke

14. NOSTALGIA 14.___
    - A. homesickness
    - B. inertia
    - C. gloominess
    - D. nasal catarrh
    - E. wanderlust

15. OCCULT 15.___
    - A. abstract
    - B. manifest
    - C. secret
    - D. oriental
    - E. acute

16. ONEROUS 16.___
    - A. unwanted
    - B. impossible
    - C. delicate
    - D. burdensome
    - E. facile

17. OPULENT 17.___
    - A. expensive
    - B. oily
    - C. crafty
    - D. profuse
    - E. jejune

18. ORDINANCE 18.___
    - A. excess weight
    - B. anarchy
    - C. law
    - D. military supplies
    - E. mound of filth

19. ORTHOGRAPHY 19.___
    - A. correct accent
    - B. choice of words
    - C. misspelling
    - D. derivation of words
    - E. clear enunciation

20. PAROCHIAL 20.___
    - A. limited in range
    - B. sacred
    - C. stubborn
    - D. objective
    - E. easily manageable

21. PEREMPTORY 21.___
    - A. trifling
    - B. compliant
    - C. arbitrary
    - D. binding
    - E. camouflaged

22. PERVADE

    A. pass along
    B. escape quietly
    C. convince at length
    D. to be diffused throughout
    E. confine

23. PERVERSITY

    A. cruelty
    B. miserliness
    C. conformity
    D. adherent
    E. frugality

24. PHLEGMATIC

    A. stolid
    B. figurative
    C. aphasic
    D. sentient
    E. substantial

25. POIGNANT

    A. melancholy
    B. soothing
    C. doubtful
    D. keen
    E. reluctant

KEYS (CORRECT ANSWERS)

1.	B	11.	A
2.	E	12.	C
3.	E	13.	B
4.	A	14.	E
5.	B	15.	B
6.	E	16.	E
7.	A	17.	E
8.	E	18.	B
9.	A	19.	C
10.	E	20.	D

21. B
22. E
23. C
24. D
25. B

TEST 4

DIRECTIONS: Each question below consists of a word printed in capital letters, followed by five words or phrases lettered A through E. Choose the lettered word or phrase that is *most nearly* OPPOSITE in meaning to the word in capital letters. *PRINT THE LETTER OF THE CORRECT ANSWER IN THE SPACE AT THE RIGHT.*

1. PRODIGIOUS
    - A. extraordinary
    - B. commonplace
    - C. profound
    - D. prehistoric
    - E. infinitesmal

   1.___

2. PUERILE
    - A. childish
    - B. mature
    - C. feverish
    - D. immaculate
    - E. pusillanimous

   2.___

3. PUNCTILIOUS
    - A. offensively frank
    - B. willing to admit blame
    - C. sarcastically polite
    - D. precise in conduct
    - E. indiscriminate

   3.___

4. RAZE
    - A. torture
    - B. erect
    - C. salvage
    - D. destroy
    - E. prorogue

   4.___

5. RECESSIVE
    - A. inclined to go back
    - B. relating to slavery
    - C. moving forward
    - D. modest
    - E. allemorphic

   5.___

6. RENEGADE
    - A. turncoat
    - B. loyalist
    - C. habitual drunkard
    - D. confirmed criminal
    - E. one who kills a king

   6.___

7. RENASCENCE
    - A. unwinding
    - B. restoration
    - C. unscrewing
    - D. detraining
    - E. perdition

   7.___

8. RESPITE
    - A. pardon
    - B. re-trial
    - C. stay
    - D. vengeance
    - E. continuation

   8.___

9. SALIENT
    - A. hidden
    - B. salty
    - C. floating
    - D. prominent
    - E. flagrant

   9.___

10. SATELLITE
    - A. falling star
    - B. attentive follower
    - C. adversary
    - D. flint spark
    - E. fellow captive

    10.___

11. SCRUPULOUS 11.____
    A. niggardly   B. abusive   C. conscientious
    D. unprincipled E. guilty

12. SINEWY 12.____
    A. callused   B. enervated   C. springy
    D. slimy   E. brawny

13. SKEPTIC 13.____
    A. agnostic   B. suave   C. ingenious
    D. credulous   E. faithful

14. SPARE 14.____
    A. forbear   B. forego   C. reserve
    D. control   E. squander

15. SPORADIC 15.____
    A. isolated   B. incessant   C. dissipated
    D. involuntary   E. discrete

KEYS (CORRECT ANSWERS)

1.	E	6.	B
2.	B	7.	E
3.	E	8.	E
4.	B	9.	A
5.	C	10.	C

11. D
12. B
13. D
14. E
15. B

ANTONYMS/OPPOSITES
EXAMINATION SECTION

DIRECTIONS FOR THIS SECTION: Each question below consists of a word printed in capital letters, followed by five words or phrases lettered A through E. Choose the lettered word or phrase that is *most nearly* OPPOSITE in meaning to the word in capital letters. *PRINT THE LETTER OF THE CORRECT ANSWER IN THE SPACE AT THE RIGHT.*

TEST 1

1. ABEYANCE A. revival B. following orders C. temporary inactivity D. adjournment E. concealment   1. ...
2. ACADEMIC A. unseasoned B. scholarly C. practical D. attainable E. superficial   2. ...
3. AFFECTATION A. histrionics B. conquetry C. shield D. airs E. ingeniousness   3. ...
4. AFFILIATE A. thread B. honor C. cut away D. associate oneself E. feign   4. ...
5. ALLEGE A. deny B. declare C. arouse D. arrest E. conjure   5. ...
6. ALLEVIATE A. moderate B. assign C. tax D. antagonize E. deceive   6. ...
7. ANIMOSITY A. hatred B. affection C. sprightliness D. animalism E. contempt   7. ...
8. APATHY A. hatred B. indifference C. policy D. cowardice E. fervor   8. ...
9. APPAL A. pierce B. apportion C. dismay D. attach E. gratify   9. ...
10. AUTHENTIC A. severe B. gracious C. mendacious D. reliable E. supreme   10. ...
11. BRISK A. large B. fragile C. alert D. flagging E. tolerant   11. ...
12. BRUSQUE A. keen B. smooth C. menacing D. quick E. abrupt   12. ...
13. CALUMNIOUS A. disastrous B. quartz-like C. laudatory E. slanderous E. querulous   13. ...
14. CANDID A. straightforward B. evasive C. profound D. pleasant E. contrite   14. ...
15. CAROUSE A. cajole B. revel C. decay D. induce E. abstain   15. ...
16. CELIBATE A. chaste B. spouseless C. pertaining to funerals D. relic E. conjugal   16. ...
17. CLEMENCY A. weather condition B. climbing plant C. type of cloud D. rigor E. mercy   17. ...
18. COMMODIOUS A. inutile B. spacious C. ordinary D. interchangeable E. useful   18. ...
19. COMPETENT A. equivalent B. compact C. adequate D. based on rivalry E. maladroit   19. ...
20. COMPLICITY A. deceit B. antipathy C. partnership in wrong D. collusion E. delight in society   20. ...
21. CONSTERNATION A. dissapointment B. dismay C. disapproval D. distrust E. intrepidity   21. ...
22. CONTAMINATE A. include B. expurgate C. pollute D. adjacent E. reflect upon   22. ...
23. CORROBORATE A. withdraw B. terminate C. disavow D. confirm E. correlate   23. ...
24. COSMIC A. funny B. vast C. greasy D. childish E. finite   24. ...
25. CRITERION A. standard B. anomaly C. judgment D. analysis E. probability   25. ...

TEST 2

1. CRUCIAL — A. pending B. conditional C. critical D. unreasonable E. unessential   1. ...
2. CULPABILITY — A. misprint B. blame C. felony D. impeccability E. whitewash   2. ...
3. DAUB — A. alarm B. delay C. depict D. stupefy E. smear   3. ...
4. DELINEATE — A. crack B. blotch C. do twice D. make of linen E. describe   4. ...
5. DEVIATING — A. conspiring B. depressing C. indirect D. unswerving E. turning   5. ...
6. DILAPIDATED — A. lonely B. integral C. ruined D. sequestered E. old-fashioned   6. ...
7. DILATORY — A. reclining B. spiteful C. expeditious D. praiseworthy E. procrastinating   7. ...
8. DISPATCH — A. curb B. argue C. send off D. mend E. receive   8. ...
9. DOCILE — A. parasitic B. ungovernable C. mournful D. teachable E. compliant   9. ...
10. DRIFT — A. meaning B. tendency C. riot D. motion E. procession   10. ...
11. DUALITY — A. unity B. falsity C. biformity D. perversity E. intactness   11. ...
12. DUBIOUS — A. questionable B. categorical C. sufficient D. pleasant to the ear E. composed   12. ...
13. DURABLE — A. flimsy B. permanent C. ugly D. timely E. callous   13. ...
14. ECCENTRIC — A. peculiar B. convergent C. ecliptic D. eclectic E. pragmatic   14. ...
15. EMBELLISH — A. defraud B. deface C. represent symbolically D. point up E. review   15. ...
16. EMBRYONIC — A. accelerated B. many-colored C. rudimentary D. undeveloped E. perfected   16. ...
17. ENIGMATIC — A. cognitive B. fraudulent C. odious D. magical E. puzzling   17. ...
18. EPIGRAMMATIC — A. pointed B. national C. ungrammatical D. scabrous E. concise   18. ...
19. FANATICISM — A. perplexity B. indifference C. endurance D. flatulence E. excessive enthusiasm   19. ...
20. FORMIDABLE — A. menacing B. conventional C. loathsome D. apprehensive E. resolute   20. ...
21. GAWKY — A. gaudy B. clumsy C. meager D. elegant E. straightforward   21. ...
22. GENESIS — A. gender B. origin C. outcome D. inception E. exodus   22. ...
23. HILARITY — A. celerity B. mirth C. despondence D. abandon E. covetousness   23. ...
24. HOSTILE — A. singular B. convincing C. poisonous D. stimulating E. amicable   24. ...
25. HYBRID — A. mongrel B. eugenic C. exaggerated D. dwarfed E. homogenous   25. ...

TEST 3

1. IMPEDIMENT — A. accusation B. hindrance C. succor D. admission E. inhibition   1. ...
2. IMPERVIOUS — A. incomparable B. impenetrable C. inhuman D. trackless D. dissoluble   2. ...
3. INCREDIBLE — A. hard to believe B. skeptical C. bad beyond correction D. indisputable D. illogical   3. ...

Test 3/4

4. INGENIOUS   A. frank B. deceitful C. ingenuous   4. ...
                    D. subversive E. clever
5. INTEGRITY   A. honesty B. opprobrium C. humor D. courage 5. ...
                    E. knowledge
6. INTIMIDATE   A. to defy B. to make afraid C. to come with- 6. ...
                    out invitation D. to weary E. to make less fearful
7. INTROSPECTION   A. bending backwards B. insertion C. performa- 7. ...
                    tion D. self examination E. extroversion
8. JOSTLE   A. trip B. elbow C. bully D. rob E. quail   8. ...
9. LAVISH   A. niggardly B. extravagant C. prodigal   9. ...
                    D. convalescent E. plain
10. LENIENCY   A. transparent substance B. stringency   10. ...
                    C. fickleness D. forbearance E. decay
11. MERCENARY   A. egoistic B. pestilential C. altruistic   11. ...
                    D. greedy E. venal
12. MEDIOCRE   A. yellow B. boundless C. ordinary E. eminent 12. ...
                    E. tiny
13. NOVELTY   A. modernism B. pseudonym C. relic D. innova- 13. ...
                    tion E. quaintness
14. OBSOLETE   A. antiquated B. polite C. neglected   14. ...
                    D. rectangular E. vernal
15. ONSLAUGHT   A. furious attack B. murder C. repulse   15. ...
                    D. adventure E. severe punishment
16. OUST   A. evict B. banish C. injure D. admit   16. ...
                    E. cry out
17. PALATABLE   A. toothsome B. savory C. soft D. intoler-   17. ...
                    able E. vindictive
18. PALLID   A. wretched B. funereal C. ghastly D. spectral 18. ...
                    E. vivid
19. PALTRY   A. consequential B. pitiable C. grandiloquent 19. ...
                    D. prevalent E. petty
20. PARABLE   A. analogy B. pattern C. phenomenon D. fable   20. ...
                    E. allegory
21. PARAPHRASE   A. restate B. convey C. reword D. articulate   21. ...
                    E. translate
22. PARCH   A. swab B. saturate C. desiccate D. sponge   22. ...
                    E. scorch
23. PATHOLOGICAL   A. morbid B. virulent C. salubrious E. diseased 23. ...
                    E. implied
24. PERMEATE   A. enfilade B. traverse C. pervade D. infil-   24. ...
                    trate E. block
25. PERPETUATE   A. obliterate B. punish C. preserve D. flourish 25. ...
                    E. enshrine

TEST 4

1. PERTINENT   A. appropriate B. awkward C. obstinate   1. ...
                    D. abusive E. irrelevant
2. PONDER   A. reflect B. hazard C. argue D. reject   2. ...
                    E. consider
3. POLLUTE   A. spread B. foul C. stain D. decontaminate   3. ...
                    E. rebut
4. POSTHUMOUS   A. hastily B. extant C. inappropriate   4. ...
                    D. happening after one's death E. unawakened

Test 4/
KEYS

5. PREDILECTION   A. maintenance B. negotiation C. investment   5. ...
                  D. inclination E. evulsion
6. PRETEXT   A. reason B. fact C. excuse D. opinion   6. ...
                  E. illusion
7. PRODIGAL   A. perturbing B. wasteful C. venal D. large   7. ...
                  E. wandering
8. REFUTE   A. disobey B. disprove C. remove D. affirm   8. ...
                  E. strike out
9. RELENTLESS   A. compassionate B. unmoved by pity C. confident 9. ...
                  D. unexciting E. graceful
10. RETICENT   A. backward B. rash C. timid D. reserved   10. ...
                  E. gushing
11. SEDENTARY   A. soothing B. calm C. migratory D. aged   11. ...
                  E. stationary
12. SKEPTICISM   A. cynicism B. simplicity C. critical state of 12. ...
                  mind D. distortion E. chariness
13. SMUG   A. uncomplaisant B. adjacent C. self-satisfied 13. ...
                  D. hazy E. cozy
14. SPASMODIC   A. continuous B. intermittent C. feverish   14. ...
                  D. gradual E. momentary
15. STILTED   A. formal B. subdued C. deprived D. archaic   15. ...
                  E. facile
16. SUCCINCT   A. superfluous B. concise C. pithy D. succu-   16. ...
                  lent E. colloquial
17. SURREPTITIOUS A. stealthy B. surprising C. authorized   17. ...
                  D. affected E. unobserved
18. SUSCEPTIBLE   A. aggressive B. impotent C. cowering   18. ...
                  D. unimpressionable E. hesitant
19. TANTRUM   A. symbol B. tranquility C. commiseration   19. ...
                  D. conundrum E. display of temper
20. TATTERS   A. finery B. gossip C. sails D. riches E. rags 20. ...

KEYS (CORRECT ANSWERS)

TEST 1		TEST 2		TEST 3		TEST 4	
1. A	11. D	1. E	11. A	1. C	11. C	1. E	11. C
2. E	12. B	2. D	12. B	2. E	12. D	2. B	12. B
3. E	13. C	3. C	13. A	3. D	13. C	3. D	13. A
4. C	14. B	4. B	14. D	4. C	14. E	4. B	14. A
5. A	15. E	5. D	15. B	5. B	15. C	5. E	15. E
6. D	16. E	6. B	16. E	6. A	16. D	6. B	16. A
7. B	17. D	7. C	17. A	7. E	17. D	7. C	17. C
8. E	18. A	8. A	18. E	8. E	18. E	8. D	18. D
9. E	19. E	9. B	19. B	9. A	19. A	9. A	19. B
10. C	20. B	10. E	20. B	10. B	20. C	10. E	20. A
	21. E		21. D		21. E		
	22. B		22. C		22. B		
	23. C		23. C		23. C		
	24. E		24. E		24. E		
	25. B		25. E		25. A		

ANTONYMS/OPPOSITES
EXAMINATION SECTION
TEST 1

DIRECTIONS: Each question below consists of a word printed in capital letters, followed by five words or phrases lettered A through E. Choose the lettered word or phrase that is *most nearly* OPPOSITE in meaning to the word in capital letters. *PRINT THE LETTER OF THE CORRECT ANSWER IN THE SPACE AT THE RIGHT.*

1. CELERITY

    A. torpor B. felicity C. fame
    D. acrimony E. temerity

2. APATHETIC

    A. stoical B. amative C. lissome
    D. finical E. redolent

3. FLACCID

    A. cold B. sterile C. brave
    D. stiff E. whimsical

4. INGENUOUS

    A. foolish B. intelligent C. wily
    D. indigent E. native

5. AMENABLE

    A. prayerful B. conciliatory C. pliant
    D. truculent E. mendacious

6. PARSIMONIOUS

    A. benevolent B. worldly C. scoffing
    D. ungrammatical E. grudging

7. INDIGENOUS

    A. caustic B. factitious C. exotic
    D. opulent E. sophisticated

8. SAPIENT

    A. distasteful B. animalistic C. ignorant
    D. jejune E. zestful

9. TENUOUS

    A. substantial B. decadent C. salubrious
    D. illogical E. slender

10. ZENITH

    A. acme B. nadir C. pentacle
    D. azimuth E. apogee

1.____
2.____
3.____
4.____
5.____
6.____
7.____
8.____
9.____
10.____

2 (#1)

11. RESTIVE

    A. overactive B. refractory C. compliant
    D. uneasy E. listless

12. ADAMANT

    A. primeval B. laudatory C. polite
    D. yielding E. intractable

13. DISCRETE

    A. continuous B. separate C. foolish
    D. tactful E. serrated

14. SANGUINE

    A. bloody B. diffident C. happy
    D. pale E. confident

15. PLACATE

    A. retaliate B. confuse C. wander
    D. nettle E. condone

16. FATUOUS

    A. inane B. stout C. witty
    D. empty E. vacuous

17. INNOCUOUS

    A. toxic B. guileful C. gullible
    D. criminal E. culpable

18. DEARTH

    A. demise B. copiousness C. nativity
    D. distaste E. lack

19. RESPITE

    A. affirmation B. intermission C. continuance
    D. colloquy E. fairness

20. LACONIC

    A. turgid B. replete C. tearful
    D. negligent E. draconic

21. ANIMADVERSION

    A. censure B. distaste C. spirituality
    D. bestiality E. approbation

22. NOISOME

    A. boisterous B. beneficial C. villous
    D. pallid E. noxious

23. EXPURGATE

    A. cleanse B. harden C. improve
    D. deflect E. smirch

24. ATAVISM

    A. progression B. favoritism C. inclination
    D. cannibalism E. reversion

25. ATTRITION

    A. appeasement B. capitulation C. wearing away
    D. calming down E. aggrandizement

KEYS (CORRECT ANSWERS)

1. A
2. B
3. D
4. C
5. D

6. A
7. C
8. C
9. A
10. B

11. C
12. D
13. A
14. B
15. D

16. C
17. A
18. B
19. C
20. A

21. E
22. B
23. E
24. A
25. E

TEST 2

DIRECTIONS: Each question below consists of a word printed in capital letters, followed by five words or phrases lettered A through E. Choose the lettered word or phrase that is *most nearly* OPPOSITE in meaning to the word in capital letters. *PRINT THE LETTER OF THE CORRECT ANSWER IN THE SPACE AT THE RIGHT*

1. FABRICATE
   - A. consume
   - B. furrow
   - C. construct
   - D. materialize
   - E. delete

2. COMMAND
   - A. mandate
   - B. consummation
   - C. correlation
   - D. commitment
   - E. supplication

3. DISSIPATE
   - A. sip
   - B. amass
   - C. disturb
   - D. outdistance
   - E. disperse

4. UNBIASED
   - A. unfair
   - B. unreasonable
   - C. uniform
   - D. equitable
   - E. disquieting

5. SATURNINE
   - A. buoyant
   - B. gloomy
   - C. aspiring
   - D. incongruous
   - E. splenetic

6. PROFITABLE
   - A. preferable
   - B. chagrined
   - C. ruinous
   - D. lucrative
   - E. profligate

7. GENERATING
   - A. generous
   - B. originating
   - C. degenerating
   - D. terminating
   - E. ingenuous

8. SANCTION
   - A. safety
   - B. performance
   - C. injunction
   - D. sanctuary
   - E. permission

9. PROBABLE
   - A. perchance
   - B. imprudent
   - C. unlikely
   - D. perilous
   - E. unsavory

10. FRUITION
    - A. exposure
    - B. harvest
    - C. frustration
    - D. neglect
    - E. attainment

2 (#2)

11. RANCOROUS   11.____
    A. benign   B. confusing   C. satiated
    D. complex   E. malicious

12. AVARICIOUS   12.____
    A. munificent   B. rapacious   C. analogous
    D. perverse   E. atonal

13. UNIQUE   13.____
    A. uniform   B. single   C. utilitarian
    D. senescent E. unitary

14. PROCURE   14.____
    A. decline   B. reap   C. forfeit
    D. effect   E. contrive

15. RAVENOUS   15.____
    A. birdlike   B. hungry   C. rancid
    D. venial   E. sated

16. INNOCUOUS   16.____
    A. mixed   B. pernicious   C. defiled
    D. harmless E. diffused

17. PERMEATE   17.____
    A. smooth   B. pulverize   C. obstruct
    D. pollute   E. penetrate

18. AXIOM   18.____
    A. adage   B. proof   C. precept
    D. dictum   E. hearsay

19. RELEVANT   19.____
    A. immaterial   B. pertinent   C. relenting
    D. capable   E. released

20. POTENT   20.____
    A. secretive   B. powerful   C. restive
    D. puissant   E. enervated

21. AMELIORATE   21.____
    A. improve   B. embitter   C. alter
    D. mellow   E. impair

22. IMPENDING   22.____
    A. pendulous   B. impeding   C. fortuitous
    D. imminent   E. looming

23. LATENT

    A. tricky   B. hidden   C. pompous
    D. overt   E. hateful

24. DISCERNMENT

    A. concern   B. obtuseness   C. distance
    D. sickness E. acumen

25. SUAVE

    A. genuine   B. captive   C. gauche
    D. bland   E. captious

KEYS (CORRECT ANSWERS)

1. A
2. E
3. B
4. A
5. A

6. C
7. D
8. C
9. C
10. C

11. A
12. A
13. A
14. C
15. E

16. B
17. C
18. E
19. A
20. E

21. B
22. C
23. D
24. B
25. C

TEST 3

DIRECTIONS: Each question below consists of a word printed in capital letters, followed by five words or phrases lettered A through E. Choose the lettered word or phrase that is *most nearly* OPPOSITE in meaning to the word in capital letters. *PRINT THE LETTER OF THE CORRECT ANSWER IN THE SPACE AT THE RIGHT.*

1. WORLDLY 1.____
   - A. trifling
   - B. secular
   - C. mundane
   - D. unworthy
   - E. impractical

2. BEG 2.____
   - A. seek
   - B. implore
   - C. convert
   - D. vaunt
   - E. donate

3. ERUDITE 3.____
   - A. impolite
   - B. learned
   - C. correct
   - D. illiterate
   - E. contrite

4. CURSORY 4.____
   - A. protracted
   - B. persistent
   - C. evanescent
   - D. superficial
   - E. gentle

5. ENIGMATIC 5.____
   - A. evident
   - B. enormous
   - C. lucid
   - D. abstruse
   - E. sphinxlike

6. PROSCRIBE 6.____
   - A. banish
   - B. condemn
   - C. diagnose poorly
   - D. transcend
   - E. prescribe

7. TURBID 7.____
   - A. limpid
   - B. muddy
   - C. moody
   - D. settled
   - E. turgid

8. PERSPICACITY 8.____
   - A. keenness
   - B. penetration
   - C. rudeness
   - D. discernment
   - E. insensibility

9. CONTIGUOUS 9.____
   - A. contagious
   - B. adjoining
   - C. intolerant
   - D. unconnected
   - E. uncontaminated

10. ASSUAGE 10.____
    - A. intensify
    - B. coagulate
    - C. alleviate
    - D. congeal
    - E. molest

2 (#3)

11. PROTAGONIST
    - A. enemy
    - B. participant
    - C. champion
    - D. protector
    - E. patron

12. VIRULENT
    - A. vehement
    - B. virtuous
    - C. deadly
    - D. reparatory
    - E. virile

13. PROLIX
    - A. tiresome
    - B. exciting
    - C. wordy
    - D. terse
    - E. pompous

14. LEVITY
    - A. lengthiness
    - B. glumness
    - C. lenience
    - D. frivolity
    - E. lewdness

15. METICULOUS
    - A. careful
    - B. approximate
    - C. untrue
    - D. metallic
    - E. indiscriminate

16. ANALOGOUS
    - A. tantamount
    - B. extracurricular
    - C. distinctive
    - D. presumptuous
    - E. cavernous

17. VICARIOUS
    - A. inconsiderate
    - B. direct
    - C. fraudulent
    - D. substitute
    - E. prestigious

18. ABROGATION
    - A. promulgation
    - B. repeal
    - C. extension
    - D. investigation
    - E. postponement

19. HOMOGENEOUS
    - A. manly
    - B. assorted
    - C. creamy
    - D. similar
    - E. parallel

20. ARRAIGN
    - A. accuse
    - B. convict
    - C. disentangle
    - D. disarrange
    - E. discharge

21. ABJURE
    - A. remove
    - B. disavow
    - C. acknowledge
    - D. imagine
    - E. entreat

22. INTESTATE
    - A. relating to inner parts
    - B. legally devised
    - C. shipped from one place to another
    - D. subject to taxation
    - E. not disposed of by will

23. ANCILLARY

    A. deterrent B. temporary C. auxiliary
    D. approved   E. additional

24. EXTRANEOUS

    A. foreign   B. accidental   C. mixed
    D. indigenous E. adventitious

25. DISPARAGE

    A. divide   B. dismiss   C. depreciate
    D. discourage E. dignify

KEYS (CORRECT ANSWERS)

1. E
2. E
3. D
4. A
5. C

6. E
7. A
8. E
9. D
10. A

11. A
12. D
13. D
14. B
15. E

16. C
17. B
18. A
19. B
20. E

21. C
22. B
23. A
24. D
25. E

TEST 4

DIRECTIONS: Each question below consists of a word printed in capital letters, followed by five words or phrases lettered A through E. Choose the lettered word or phrase that is *most nearly* OPPOSITE in meaning to the word in capital letters. *PRINT THE LETTER OF THE CORRECT ANSWER IN THE SPACE AT THE RIGHT.*

1. FUGACIOUS
   - A. pugnacious
   - B. tenacious
   - C. mendacious
   - D. settled
   - E. migratory

2. THRASONICAL
   - A. treasonable
   - B. gingival
   - C. vainglorious
   - D. unassuming
   - E. lyrical

3. PELAGIC
   - A. terrestrial
   - B. aquatic
   - C. noncontagious
   - D. polemical
   - E. epigrammatic

4. FUSCOUS
   - A. importunate
   - B. chaste
   - C. radiant
   - D. fractious
   - E. amenable

5. CREPUSCULAR
   - A. glimmering
   - B. crackling
   - C. pussy
   - D. mutable
   - E. distinct

6. NOISOME
   - A. attractive
   - B. noxious
   - C. inoffensive
   - D. winsome
   - E. noiseless

7. PEJORATIVE
   - A. appreciative
   - B. acceding
   - C. ultimate
   - D. alliterative
   - E. conceding

8. JEJUNE
   - A. valiant
   - B. vital
   - C. graceful
   - D. senile
   - E. incipient

9. FULGENT
   - A. divergent
   - B. lambent
   - C. unresplendent
   - D. cogent
   - E. indigent

10. LENITIVE
    - A. laxative
    - B. provocative
    - C. menial
    - D. incursive
    - E. malevolent

11. IRREFRAGABLE

    A. breakable   B. desirable   C. tractable
    D. inconclusive E. refutable

12. INCHOATE

    A. chaotic   B. disclosed   C. coherent
    D. infatuated   E. complete

13. MINATORY

    A. vanishing   B. nugatory   C. myriad
    D. malignant   E. propitious

14. AMBIENT

    A. wandering   B. pandering   C. transient
    D. remote   E. hostile

15. EUPHEMISTIC

    A. euphuistic   B. grating   C. masochistic
    D. palpable   E. insolent

16. FACTIOUS

    A. fractious   B. fictitious   C. scrupulous
    D. seemly   E. disinterested

17. FRIABLE

    A. unseasoned   B. palatable   C. renascent
    D. indestructible E. adhesive

18. HEGEMONY

    A. thraldom   B. testimony   C. followership
    D. necromancy   E. obligation

19. IMMANENT

    A. illative   B. imminent   C. emanating
    D. unessential E. clement

20. INDEFEASIBLE

    A. defensible   B. abrogable   C. disputable
    D. deferential E. execrable

21. EQUIVOCAL

    A. ambiguous   B. ambivalent   C. equitable
    D. esoteric   E. unquestionable

22. LIVID

    A. lurid   B. discolored   C. unrestrained
    D. rubicund   E. ghastly

23. MOIETY

    A. impiety
    B. notoriety
    C. unity
    D. harmony
    E. inconsistency

24. PEREMPTORY

    A. dogmatic
    B. authoritarian
    C. indecisive
    D. conciliatory
    E. whimsical

25. VENIAL

    A. mercenary
    B. venous
    C. purulent
    D. aberrant
    E. loathsome

23. ___
24. ___
25. ___

KEYS (CORRECT ANSWERS)

1. D
2. D
3. A
4. C
5. E
6. C
7. A
8. B
9. C
10. B
11. E
12. E
13. E
14. D
15. B
16. E
17. D
18. A
19. D
20. B
21. E
22. D
23. C
24. C
25. E

ARITHMETIC

EXAMINATION SECTION
TEST 1

DIRECTIONS: Each question or incomplete statement is followed by several suggested answers or completions. Select the one that BEST answers the question or completes the statement. *PRINT THE LETTER OF THE CORRECT ANSWER IN THE SPACE AT THE RIGHT.*

1. 215 x 30 =
    A. 650
    B. 6450
    C. 6500
    D. None of the above

2. How much is saved by buying a $60 bicycle for cash instead of paying $5.25 a month for a year?
    A. $3.00
    B. $6.00
    C. $7.50
    D. None of the above

3. How many square inches are in a square foot?
    A. 12
    B. 24
    C. 144
    D. None of the above

4. What is ten thousand multiplied by one thousand?
    A. One hundred thousand
    B. One million
    C. Ten million
    D. None of the above

5. $4\ 1/6 + 3\ 1/12 =$
    A. $7\frac{1}{4}$
    B. $7\frac{7}{12}$
    C. $8\frac{1}{4}$
    D. None of the above

6. Tom is awake an average of 15 hours each day. How many hours does he sleep in a week?
    A. 9
    B. 45
    C. 105
    D. None of the above

7. If peppermints costing 70¢ per lb. come in 1 1/2 lb. boxes, what is the cost of 5 boxes?
    A. $3.50
    B. $5.25
    C. $5.75
    D. None of the above

8. What is 349,638 rounded to the nearest hundred?
    A. 349,600
    B. 349,640
    C. 350,000
    D. None of the above

9. 6 1/9 - 3 1/3 =

    A. 2 7/9   B. 2 8/9
    C. 3 1/2   D. None of the above

10. Which is less than one-thousandth of an inch?

    A. .025 in.   B. .004 in.
    C. .0008 in.   D. None of the above

11. Which is ten million three thousand?

    A. 10,300,000   B. 10,030,000
    C. 10,003,000   D. None of the above

12. $\frac{1}{2} + \frac{1}{3} + \frac{1}{6}$

    A. $\frac{1}{11}$ B. $\frac{5}{6}$
    C. 1   D. None of the above

13. 2/5 of 20 =

    A. 1/8   B. 8
    C. 50   D. None of the above

14. In the following multiplication, N stands for a number.

    4N5
      4
    ―――
    1740

    What is the number?

    A. 3   B. 6
    C. 8   D. None of the above

15. 7/8 - 1/2

    A. 3/8   B. 3/4
    C. 1   D. None of the above

16. The scale for a house plan is 1/4 in. =1 ft.
How long is a hall that is 3 inches long on the plan?

    A. 7 ft.   B. $12\frac{1}{2}$ ft.
    C. 16 ft.   D. None of the above

17. 4 1/5 x 1 3/7 =

    A. 5   B. 5 22/35
    C. 6   D. None of the above

18. 7/3 - 11/6

    A. 1/2
    B. 1 3/11
    C. 1 1/3
    D. None of the above

19. The school pool is 60 feet long.
    How many lengths must John swim to pass his 100-yard swimming test?

    A. 2
    B. 5
    C. 6
    D. None of the above

20. A store bought a dozen clocks for $72 and sold each for 50% more than it cost. What was the selling price of one clock?

    A. $6.50
    B. $9.00
    C. $26.00
    D. None of the above

21. If J stands for John's age and F for his father's age, which shows that John is 26 years younger than his father?

    A. J + F = 26
    B. J - 26 = F
    C. J + 26 = F
    D. None of the above

22. The board at the right has five equally spaced holes. What is the distance between the centers of holes 2 and 3?
    A. 8"
    B. 10"
    C. 20"
    D. None of the above

    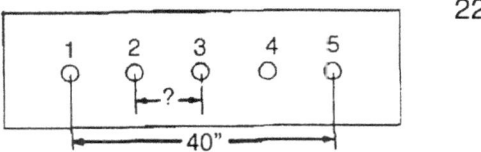

23. $.07 \overline{)51.1} =$

    A. 7.3
    B. 73
    C. 730
    D. None of the above

24. Joe worked from 8:30 A.M. until 4:45 P.M., except for 45 minutes for lunch. How many hours did he work?

    A. $6\frac{1}{2}$
    B. $7\frac{1}{2}$
    C. $8\frac{1}{2}$
    D. None of the above

25. A highway 150 miles long cost $130 million. What was the AVERAGE cost per mile?

    A. Between $12,000 and $13,000
    B. Between $200,000 and $300,000
    C. Between $800,000 and $900,000
    D. None of the above

KEY (CORRECT ANSWERS)

1. B
2. A
3. C
4. C
5. A

6. D
7. B
8. A
9. A
10. C

11. C
12. C
13. B
14. A
15. A

16. D
17. C
18. A
19. B
20. B

21. C
22. B
23. C
24. B
25. C

SOLUTIONS TO PROBLEMS

1. $(215)(30) = 6450$

2. Savings = $(\$5.25)(12) - \$60 = \$3.00$

3. $(12)(12) = 144$ sq.in. $= 1$ sq.ft.

4. $(10,000)(1000) = 10,000,000 =$ ten million

5. $4\frac{1}{6} + 3\frac{1}{12} = 4\frac{2}{12} + 3\frac{1}{12} = 7\frac{3}{12} = 7\frac{1}{4}$

6. $(9)(7) = 63$ hours of sleep per week

7. $(5)(1\frac{1}{2})(.70) = \$5.25$

8. $349,638 = 349,600$ when rounded to the nearest hundred

9. $6\frac{1}{9} - 3\frac{1}{3} = 6\frac{1}{9} - 3\frac{3}{9} = 5\frac{10}{9} - 3\frac{3}{9} = 2\frac{7}{9}$

10. .0008 in. is less than .001 in.

11. $10,003,000 =$ ten million three thousand

12. $\frac{1}{2} + \frac{1}{3} + \frac{1}{6} = \frac{3}{6} + \frac{2}{6} + \frac{1}{6} = 1$

13. $(\frac{2}{5})(\frac{20}{1}) = \frac{40}{5} = 8$

14. If N = 3, we have $(435)(4) = 1740$. Note: $(5)(4) = 0$ digit and a carry-over of 2 in this multiplication. So, $4 \times N + 2 = 1$ digit Only N = 3 or N = 8 would fit. But note that the final answer of 1740 would eliminate 8 as a choice.

15. $\frac{7}{8} - \frac{1}{2} = \frac{7}{8} - \frac{4}{8} = \frac{3}{8}$

16. $3'' \div \frac{1}{4} = 12$. Then, $(12)(1 \text{ ft.}) = 12$ ft.

17. $4\frac{1}{5} \times 1\frac{3}{7} = (\frac{21}{5})(\frac{10}{7}) = \frac{210}{35} = 6$

18. $\frac{7}{3} - \frac{11}{6} = \frac{14}{6} - \frac{11}{6} = \frac{3}{6} = \frac{1}{2}$

19. 100 yds. = 300 ft. Then, 300 ÷ 60 = 5 lengths

20. $72 ÷ 12 = $6.00. Then, ($6.00)(1.50) = $9.00

21. J + 26 = F shows that John is 26 years younger than his father.

22. The distance from hole 1 to hole 5 = 40", so the distance between any two consecutive holes = 40" ÷ 4 = 10"

23. 51.1 ÷ .07 = 730

24. From 8:30 AM to 4:45 PM = 8¼ hrs. Then, hrs. of 3 work. (Note: 45 min. = 3/4 hr.)

25. $130,000,000 ÷ 150 = = $866,666.67 average cost per mile.

    This figure is between $800,000 and $900,000.

TEST 2

DIRECTIONS: Each question or incomplete statement is followed by several suggested answers or completions. Select the one that BEST answers the question or completes the statement. *PRINT THE LETTER OF THE CORRECT ANSWER IN THE SPACE AT THE RIGHT.*

1. What is the volume of the box shown at the right?
   A. 7 cu. ft.
   B. 12 cu. ft.
   C. 14 cu. ft.
   D. None of the above

   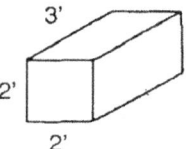

   1.____

2. If lemonade is made by mixing 1 pint of lemon juice with 3 quarts of water, how much lemon juice should be mixed with 3 gallons of water?

   A. 2 quarts
   B. 3 quarts
   C. 1 gallon
   D. None of the above

   2.____

3. What is the area of the figure shown at the right?
   A. 3 sq. in.
   B. 5 sq. in.
   C. 10 sq. in.
   D. None of the above

   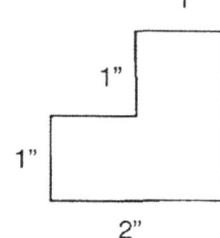

   3.____

4. $\dfrac{21 \times 14 \times 30}{28 \times 15 \times 7} =$

   A. 2
   B. 3
   C. 21
   D. None of the above

   4.____

5. 125% of 60 =

   A. 75
   B. 750
   C. 7500
   D. None of the above

   5.____

6. In the formula I = .05pt, I is the interest due on p dollars borrowed at 5% for t years. What is I if p = $500?

   A. 25t
   B. .10t
   C. .05(500+t)
   D. None of the above

   6.____

7. 4 x 6 = ? x 8. ? =

   A. 3
   B. 24
   C. 192
   D. None of the above

   7.____

8. On a day in January, the temperature in Central City was -18° F. How many degrees below freezing was this?

   A. 14
   B. 18
   C. 50
   D. None of the above

   8.____

9. .875 =

   A. $\dfrac{875}{100}$
   B. $\dfrac{5}{8}$
   C. 7 / 2
   D. None of the above

10. What is the area of the right triangle shown at the right?
    A. 6 sq. ft.
    B. 12 sq. ft.
    C. 60 sq. ft.
    D. None of the above

11. A United States Savings Bond costs $18.75. How many can be bought for $150?
    A. 6
    B. 8
    C. 12
    D. None of the above

12. One half of a melon was divided equally among 4 boys. What portion of the whole melon did each boy get?
    A. 1/8
    B. 1/6
    C. 1/4
    D. None of the above

13. One third of a foot is what part of a yard?
    A. 1/6
    B. 1/9
    C. 1/12
    D. None of the above

14. What is the sum of XXVIII and XII?
    A. D
    B. XC
    C. XL
    D. None of the above

15. How many people can each have pint of punch from one gallon of punch?
    A. 8
    B. 16
    C. 32
    D. None of the above

16. How much are license plates for a car weighing 3500 lbs. if the cost is $.50 per 100 lbs.?
    A. $17.50
    B. $35.00
    C. $70.00
    D. None of the above

17. What percent of the figure is black?
    A. 20%
    B. 25%
    C. 33 1/3%
    D. None of the above

18. Each week, Bill saves $2 of his own money and $3 given him by his father. When the total is $25, how much of it was from Bill's own money?
    A. $10.00
    B. $12.50
    C. $20.00
    D. None of the above

19. $\dfrac{3}{8} \div \dfrac{1}{4}$

    A. 25   B. .5
    C. 1.5   D. None of the above

20. If the price of a $5 tablecloth is reduced by $1, what is the percent reduction?

    A. 4%   B. 20%
    C. 25%   D. None of the above

KEY (CORRECT ANSWERS)

1.	B	11.	B
2.	A	12.	A
3.	A	13.	B
4.	B	14.	C
5.	A	15.	B
6.	A	16.	A
7.	A	17.	B
8.	C	18.	A
9.	C	19.	C
10.	A	20.	B

SOLUTIONS TO PROBLEMS

1. Volume = (2')(2')(3') = 12 cu.ft.

2. 3 gallons = 12 qts. and 12 qts. 3 qts. = 4.
   Thus, (1 pt)(4) = 4 pts = 2 qts of lemon juice.

3. 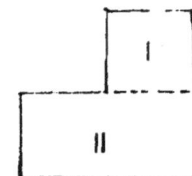 Area of I = 1" x 1" = 1 sq.in.
   Area of II = 2" x 1" = 2 sq.in.
   Total area = 3 sq.in.

4. $[(21)(14)(30)] \div [(28)(15)(7)] = 8820 \div 2940 = 3$

5. (1.25)(60) = 75

6. I = (.05)($500)(t) = 25t

7. 4 x 6 = 24. Then, 24 ÷ 8 = 3

8. -18°F = 32° - (-18°) = 50° below freezing

9. $.875 = \frac{875}{1000} = \frac{7}{8}$

10. Area = (1/2)(3')(4') = 6 sq.ft.

11. $150 ÷ $18.75 = 8 bonds

12. $\frac{1}{2} \div 4 = \frac{1}{2} \times \frac{1}{4} = \frac{1}{8}$ melon

13. $\frac{1}{3} \text{ft} = (\frac{1}{3})(12") = 4"$ and $\frac{4"}{36"} = \frac{1}{9}$ yd.

14. XXVIII + XII = 28 + 12 = 40 = XL

15. 1 gallon = 8 pints. 8 Pints ÷ $\frac{1}{2}$ Pint = 16 servings

16. 3500 ÷ 100 = 35, so (35)($.50) = $17.50

17. $\frac{3}{12}$ = 25% of these boxes are black

18. Let x = Bill's own money. Then, $\frac{2}{5} = \frac{x}{25}$ Solving, x = $10

19. $\frac{3}{8} \div \frac{1}{4} = (\frac{3}{8})(\frac{4}{1}) = \frac{12}{8} = 1.5$

20. $\frac{1}{5}$ = 20% reduction

EXAMINATION SECTION

TEST 1

DIRECTIONS: Each question or incomplete statement is followed by several suggested answers or completions. Select the one that BEST answers the question or completes the statement. *PRINT THE LETTER OF THE CORRECT ANSWER IN THE SPACE AT THE RIGHT.*

1. 2/3 × 12 equals
   A. 4
   B. 6
   C. 8
   D. 18
   E. None of the above

   1.____

2. 83.97
   1.78
   14.36
   9.03
   The sum of the above column is
   A. 99.13   B. 99.24   C. 109.14   D. 109.23   E. 109.24

   2.____

3. The value of x in the equation 5x = 75 is
   A. 13
   B. 15
   C. 70
   D. 80
   E. None of the above

   3.____

4. 65 ÷ .13 equals
   A. .501
   B. 5.01
   C. 50.1
   D. 501
   E. None of the above

   4.____

5. The sum of 6 feet 8 inches and 3 feet 4 inches is
   A. 2 ft. 2 in.
   B. 9 ft.
   C. 10 ft.
   D. 10 ft. 12 in.
   E. None of the above

   5.____

6. 3/4 – 1/2 + 1/8 equals
   A. 3/10
   B. 3/8
   C. 5/8
   D. 1 3/8
   E. None of the above

   6.____

7. 4 5/16 – 2 3/8 equals
   A. 1 15/16
   B. 2 1/16
   C. 2 ¼
   D. 2 15/16
   E. None of the above

   7.____

8. (-12)+(-3) equals
   A. -9
   B. +15
   C. +9
   D. -15
   E. None of the above

   8.____

9. The ratio of the lengths of two lines is 5 to 3. The length of the shorter line is 30 inches. The length of the longer line is _____ inches.
   A. 18
   B. 48
   C. 50
   D. 140
   E. None of the above

   9.____

10. .025 written as a common fraction is
    A. 25/10
    B. 25/100
    C. 25/1000
    D. 25/10,000
    E. None of the above

    10.____

11. In the proportion 5/2 = 9/x the value of x is
    A. 1.8
    B. 3.6
    C. 22.5
    D. 36
    E. None of the above

    11.____

12. 33 1/3 percent of 3 equals
    A. 1
    B. 10
    C. 100/3
    D. 100
    E. None of the above

    12.____

13. $\sqrt{233}$ equals
    A. 15
    B. 20.5
    C. 25
    D. 112.5
    E. None of the above

    13.____

14. On the portion of the scale shown at the right, the reading to which the arrow points is _____ units.
    A. 6 3/16
    B. 6 3/5
    C. 6 3/4
    D. 7 5/8
    E. None of the above

    14.____

15. If 4x/5 − 6 = 10, then x equals
    A. 15 1/5
    B. 5
    C. 4
    D. 3 1/5
    E. None of the above

    15.____

16. The difference between 8 hours 0 minutes 6 seconds and 6 hours 4 minutes 15 seconds is _____ hr. _____ min. _____ seconds.
    A. 0; 54; 51
    B. 1; 54; 51
    C. 2; 4; 9
    D. 2; 54; 45
    E. None of the above

    16.____

17. The scores made by nine pupils on a science test are: 2, 4, 6, 6, 8, 10, 12, 14, 19.
    The MEAN score is
    A. 6
    B. 8
    C. 9
    D. 81
    E. None of the above

    17.____

18. A certain cost formula is represented graphically in the figure at the right. From the graph, when n = 7, the value of C is about
    A. 140
    B. 120
    C. 110
    D. 102
    E. None of the above

    18.____

19. A simplified form of the expression A = 1/2 bh + 1/2 ah is
    A. A = ½ h(b+a)   B. bh + ah   C. A = abh
    D. $\frac{A}{1/2bh}$ = 1/2 ah   E. None of the above

19._____

20. The ratio of 6 inches to 3 feet is
    A. 6/1   B. 2/1   C. 1/2
    D. 1/18   E. None of the above

20._____

21. The value of s in the equation 3s = 12 – s is
    A. 6   B. 4   C. 3 2/3
    D. 3   E. None of the above

21._____

22. 16 2/3 percent of what number is 30?
    A. 5   B. 18   C. 160
    D. 180   E. None of the above

22._____

23. The line graph shown at the right represents the temperature readings in Albany, New York, at two-hour intervals from 4 A.M. to 10 P.M. on a certain day in February. The APPROXIMATE change in temperature between 7 A.M. and 9 A.M. is _____ degrees.
    A. 3.5
    B. 3.0
    C. 2.5
    D. 2.0
    E. None of the above

23._____

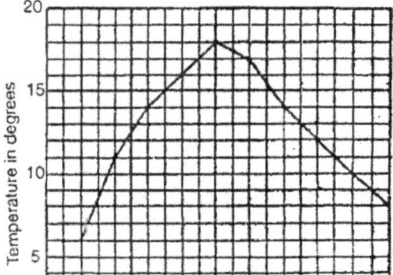

Questions 24-25.

DIRECTIONS: Questions 24 and 25 are to be answered on the basis of the following figure and information.

In the figure below, a square whose side is b is cut from a square whose side is a.

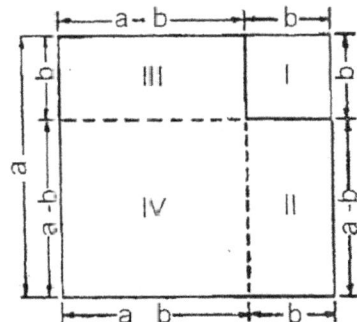

24. The sum of the perimeters of Section I and Section III can be represented by   24.____
    A. b^2 B. $4a - 2b$ C. $2a + 3b$
    D. $a(a-b)$ E. None of the above

25. The sum of the areas of Section II and Section IV can be represented by   25.____
    A. b^2 B. $4a - 2b$ C. $2a + 3b$
    D. $a(a-b)$ E. None of the above

26. The temperature reading (F) on the Fahrenheit scale equals 32 more than   26.____
    9/5 of the Centigrade reading (C).
    This rule when translated into symbols is expressed by
    A. F = 9/5C + 32   B. F = 9/5(C+32)   C. F = 9/5 + 32C
    D. F + 32 = 9/5C   E. None of the above

27. In the equation 6x – 114 = .3x, the value of x is   27.____
    A. 38   B. 20   C. 12 2/3
    D. 2   E. None of the above

28. What percent of 42 is 84?   28.____
    A. 4%   B. 2%   C. 50%
    D. 200%   E. None of the above

29. The CORRECT name of the solid figure at the   29.____
    right is
       A. semicircle
       B. circle
       C. sphere
       D. cone
       E. cylinder

30. Which of these fractions has the LARGEST value?   30.____
    A. 1/2   B. 5/9   C. 7/12
    D. 2/3   E. 3/4

31. The formula for the area of a circle is A =   31.____
    A. π^2 B. $2/3\,\pi^2$ C. $2\pi r$
    D. bh   E. None of the above

32. The CORRECT name of the figure at the right is   32.____
       A. pentagon
       B. hexagon
       C. rectangle
       D. trapezoid
       E. square

112

33. The figure at the right is a
    A. rectangle
    B. square
    C. pentagon
    D. trapezoid
    E. parallelogram

33.____

34. If x = -18, y = 3, and z = -2, then x − y + z equals
    A. 3   B. -3   C. -23   D. -52   E. -56

34.____

35. The number 335,560 rounded off to the nearest thousand is
    A. 335,000   B. 335,500   C. 336,000
    D. 340,000   E. None of the above

35.____

36. In the triangle ABC at the right, the sum of the angles is _____ degrees
    A. 360
    B. 180
    C. 90
    D. 35
    E. None of the above

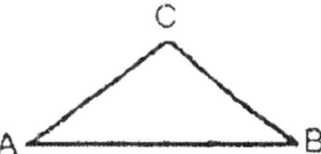

36.____

37. According to the map shown at the right, the APPROXIMATE distance between the southern point of New York City and Albany is _____ miles.
    A. 50
    B. 75
    C. 130
    D. 180
    E. 200

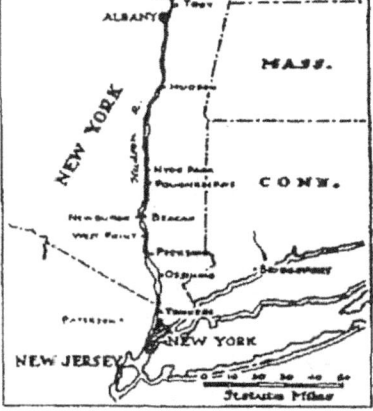

37.____

38. If 6 is added to a certain number n, the result is 1. An equation which expresses this relationship is
    A. n + 6 = 1   B. n − 1 = 6   C. 6 − n = 1
    D. n + 1 = 6   E. None of the above

38.____

39. In the expression $2n^3$, the 3 is called a(n)
    A. coefficient   B. factor   C. exponent
    D. multiplicand   E. None of the above

39.____

40. The number of inches in n feet is represented by
    A. 12n   B. 3n   C. n/3
    D. n/12   E. None of the above

40.____

41. The simple interest on $600 for 3 months at 4 percent per year is represented by 600 × .04x
    A. 1/4
    B. 1/3
    C. 3
    D. 4
    E. None of the above

41._____

42. The circle graph shown at the right indicates how a family's annual budget of $3,000 was planned.
    Food   40 percent
    Shelter   25 percent
    Clothes   15 percent
    Operating Expenses 10 percent
    Insurance & Savings 10 percent
    The part of the circle representing Shelter is _____ degrees.
    A. 25
    B. 45
    C. 90
    D. 250
    E. None of the above

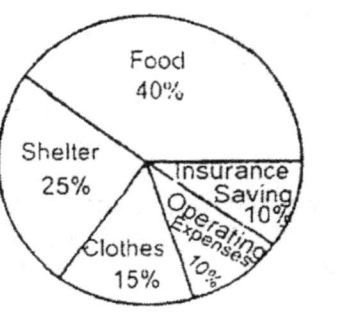

42._____

43. In the parallelogram ABCD shown at the right, each small square represents 4 square inches. The area of the right triangle AED represents _____ square inches.
    A. 3
    B. 12
    C. 24
    D. 48
    E. None of the above

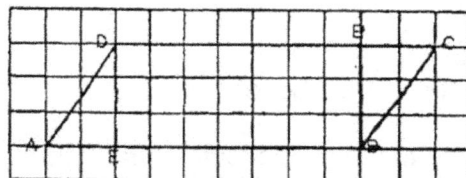

45._____

44. A surveyor measured angle x with a transit. (See figure at the right.) Angle x is called
    A. the angle of depression B from A
    B. an obtuse angle
    C. the supplement of angle
    D. the angle of elevation of B from A
    E. none of the above

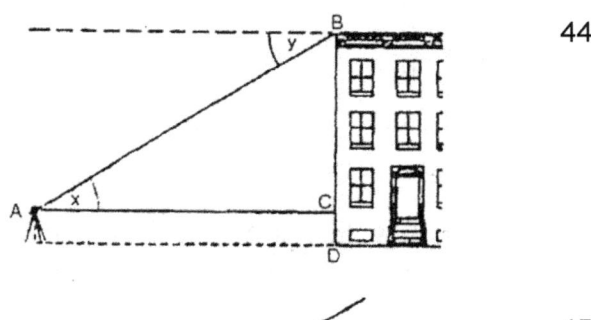

44._____

45. In the figure at the right, AOB is a straight line. An equation showing the relationship between u and v is
    A. u = 1/2v
    B. u = 180 – v
    C. u + v = 90
    D. v = 3u
    E. None of the above

45._____

46. If x = 4 when y = 6 and x varies directly as y, then when y = 15, x equals
    A. 20   B. 10   C. 1 3/5
    D. 1 1/3   E. None of the above

47. A discount of 15 percent from a marked price produces a net price which is _____ of the marked price.
    A. .15%   B. .85%   C. 15%   D. 85%   E. 115%

48. When the formula $A = P + Prt$ is solved for t, t equals
    A. $A - P - Pr$ B. $\frac{A-Pr}{P}$ C. $\frac{A-P}{1+r}$
    D. $\frac{A-P}{Pr}$ E. None of the above

49. The Greek letter π
    A. was assigned the value 3.1416 by the International Court of Law
    B. was given an arbitrary value of 22/7 by a famous mathematician
    C. was discovered to be exactly 3.142
    D. when multiplied by the radius of a circle equals the area
    E. is used as a symbol for the ratio of the circumference of a circle to its diameter

50. If the base and altitude of a triangle are doubled, the area
    A. remains constant   B. is multiplied by 4   C. is doubled
    D. is divided by 4   E. is none of the above

51. Each side of the equilateral triangle in the figure at the right is s inches long. The length of an altitude of the triangle is represented as
    A. s in.
    B. $s\sqrt{2}$
    C. $s\sqrt{3}$
    D. $\frac{s\sqrt{3}}{2}$ in.
    E. None of the above

52. The length of a meter is about _____ inches.
    A. 1   B. 6   C. 12   D. 40   E. 100

53. A point which lies on the straight-line graph of the equation $2x - 3y = 12$ is
    A. (3,-2)   B. (2,-3)   C. (-4,0)
    D. (0,6)   E. None of the above

54. If the two parallel lines AB and CD in the figure at the right are cut by a third line, EF, then the FALSE statement is
   A. ∠r + ∠s = ∠s + ∠y
   B. ∠y + ∠w = ∠t + ∠s
   C. ∠u + ∠w = ∠s + ∠x
   D. ∠r + ∠x = ∠t + ∠w
   E. ∠s + ∠u = ∠r + ∠t

55. The product of n^4 and n^2 equals
   A. $2n^8$ B. $2n^6$ C. n^8
   D. n^2 E. None of the above

56. The volume of the rectangular solid shown at the right is
   A. 12 cu. in.
   B. 44 sq. in.
   C. 48 cu. in.
   D. 88 sq. in.
   E. None of the above

57. Baseball bats listed at twenty-one dollars per dozen are sold to schools at a discount of 20 percent.
   How much do they cost the schools per dozen?
   A. $4.20   B. $16.80   C. $20.80
   D. $25.20   E. None of the above

58. Last year a Chicago merchant's total business amounted to $30,000. For the goods sold, he paid $12,000, for rent he paid $2,500, for clerk services $4,742, and for other expenses $1,058.
   His average monthly net profit was
   A. $676.67   B. $891.67   C. $2,500.00
   D. $9,700.00   E. None of the above

59. If the marked price of an article is $100 and the first discount is 10 percent and the second discount 2 percent, the sale price is
   A. $78.20   B. $88.00   C. $88.20
   D. $88.80   E. None of the above

60. Mr. Smith agreed to pay an automobile agency a commission of 18 percent of the selling price of his car.
   If the selling price was $1,250, Mr. Smith would receive
   A. $225.00   B. $1,025.00   C. $1,227.50
   D. $1,475.00   E. None of the above

61. Mr. Browne receives $30.45 per year on an investment of $870.
   At this rate, if his total investment was $1,500, his annual interest would be
   A. $52.50   B. $62.50   C. $625.00
   D. $655.45   E. None of the above

62. The Ephrata National Bank discounted a 60-day note for $3,500 at 3½ percent per year.
    The proceeds of the note were
    A. $3,377.50 B. $3,479.58 C. $3,520.42
    D. $3,622.50 E. None of the above

    62.____

63. The normal weight of an adult can be found by using the formula w = 5.5(20+d), where w represents the weight in pounds and d the number of inches one's height exceeds 5 feet.
    By this formula, the normal weight of an adult who is 5'6" tall is _____ pounds.
    A. 134 B. 140.25 C. 140.8
    D. 143.0 E. None of the above

    63.____

64. In the figure at the right, triangles ACB and ADE are similar triangles   The length of side DE is _____ feet.
    A. 30
    B. 32
    C. 48
    D. 50
    E. None of the above

    64.____

65. A square piece of tin shown in the figure at the right is used to make an open box. One-inch squares are cut from each corner of the piece of tin and the sides then turned up, to form a box containing 49 cubic inches.
    The length of a side of the original square piece of tin required to make this box is _____ inches.
    A. 5
    B. 7
    C. 8
    D. 9
    E. None of the above

    65.____

KEY (CORRECT ANSWERS)

1. C	11. B	21. D	31. A	41. A	51. D	61. A
2. C	12. A	22. D	32. A	42. C	52. D	62. B
3. B	13. A	23. C	33. E	43. B	53. A	63. D
4. D	14. E	24. E	34. C	44. D	54. E	64. B
5. C	15. E	25. D	35. C	45. B	55. E	65. D
6. B	16. E	26. A	36. B	46. B	56. C	
7. A	17. C	27. B	37. C	47. D	57. B	
8. D	18. A	28. D	38. A	48. D	58. E	
9. C	19. A	29. E	39. C	49. E	59. C	
10. C	20. E	30. E	40. A	50. B	60. B	

11 (#1)

SOLUTIONS TO PROBLEMS

1. $2/3 \times 12 = \frac{12}{1} = \frac{24}{3} = 8$

2. Adding, we get 109.14

3. If 5x = 75, x = 75/5 = 15

4. 65.13 ÷ 13 = 501

5. 6 ft. 8 in. + 3 ft. 4 in. = 9 ft. 12 in. = 10 ft.

6. 3/4 – 1/2 + 1/8 = 6/8 – 4/8 + 1/8 = 3/8

7. 4 15/16 – 2 3/8 = 3 21/16 – 2 6/16 = 1 15/16

8. (-12) + (-3) = -15

9. Let x = length of longer line. Then, 5:3 = x:30. Solving, x = 50

10. .025 = 25/1000 (Can also be reduced to 1/40)

11. Cross-multiplying, 5x = 18. Thus, 18/5 = 3.6

12. 33 1/3% of 3 = (1/3)(3) = 1

13. $\sqrt{225}$ = 15, since 15^2 = 225

14. The arrow points to 6 3/8

15. 4x/5 – 6 = 10. Adding 6, 4x/5 = 16. Then, x = 16 ÷ 4/5 = 20

16. 8 hrs. 0 min. 6 sec. – 6 hrs. 4 min. 15 sec. can be written as 7 hrs. 59 min. 66 sec. – 6 hrs. 4 min. 15 sec. to get 1 hr. 55 min. 51 sec.

17. Mean = (2+4+6+8+10+12+14+19) ÷ 9 = 9

18. When n = 0, c = 0. When n = 5, c = 100. Thus, c = 20n. Finally, for n = 7, c = (20)(7) = 140

19. A = 1/2 bh + 1/2 h(b+a)

20. 6 inches : 3 feet = 6 inches : 36 inches = 1/6

21. Add 5 to both sides to get 4s = 12, so s = 3

22. 16 2/3% of x is 30. Then, 1/6 x = 30. Then, 1/6 x = 180

12 (#1)

23. At 7:00 A.M. the temperature was 12.5, while at 9:00 A.M. the temperature was 15. The change was 2.5 degrees.

24. Perimeter of Section I is 4b and the perimeter of Section III is 2b + 2a – 2b = 2a. The sum of the perimeters is 4b + 2a.

25. Area of Section II is b(a-b) = ab – b^2 and the area of Section IV is $(a-b)^2 = a^2 - 2ab + b^2$. The sum of the areas is $a^2 - ab = a(a-b)$.

26. Direct translation of words to symbols yields F = 9/5C + 32

27. Subtract 6x to get -114 = 5.7x. Solving, x = 20

28. (84/42)(100)% = 200%

29. The figure is a cylinder.

30. Converting each choice to a decimal, we get .5, .$\overline{5}$, .58$\overline{3}$, .6, .75. The largest is .75 corresponding to 3/4.

31. For a circle, A = πr^2

32. A five-sided enclosed figure with straight sides is called a pentagon.

33. A quadrilateral with opposite sides parallel is called a parallelogram. Rectangles and squares are parallelograms with 90° angles.

34. x – y + z = 18 – 3 – 2 = 23

35. Since the digit in the hundreds place is 5 or greater, the answer is 336,000.

36. The sum of the angles of any triangle is 180°.

37. The scale difference is about 2 inches, and since 50 miles corresponds to 3/4 inch, the actual distance is about (50)(2÷3/4) = 133 1/3 mi. Closest answer given s 130 mi.

38. 6 added to n means 6 + n. Thus, 6 + n = 1 or n + 6 = 1.

39. 3 is an exponent for $2n^3$.

40. 12 inches in 1 foot means 12n inches in n feet.

41. 3 months = 1/4 year

42. 25% of 360 degrees = 90 degrees.

43. Area of △AED = (1/2)(2)(3) = 3 square units = 12 sq. inches.

44. Angle X is the angle of elevation to B from A.

13 (#1)

45. Since u + v = 180, we can also write u = 180 − v

46. 4/x = 6/15 Cross-multiplying, 6x = 60. Solving, x = 10

47. 100% − 15% = 85%

48. A = P + Prt becomes A − P = Prt. Dividing by Pr, we get: t = (A−P)/Pr

49. π = ratio of circumference to diameter of a circle.

50. Let B = base, H = altitude. Original area of triangle = 1/2BH. If new base and altitude are 2B and 2H, new area = ½(2B)(2H) = 2BH, which is 4 times the value of 1/2BH.

51. Let x = altitude. Then, $x^2 + (s/2)^2 = s^2$. This becomes $3/4 s^2 = x^2$. Solving, x = s √3 /2

52. 1 meter ≈ 39.37 inches ≈ 40 inches.

53. Substituting (3,−2), 2(3) − 3(−2) = 12. The other points do not lie on 2x − 3y = 12.

54. The false statement is ∠2 + ∠u = ∠r + ∠t. It is only true that ∠x = ∠u and ∠r = ∠t).

55. $n^4 \cdot n^2 = n^6$, since exponents are added in multiplication.

56. Volume = (6)(4)(2) = 48 cu. in.

57. ($21)(.80) = $16.80

58. $30,000 − $12,000 − $2,500 − $4,742 − $1,058 = $9,700. The monthly amount is $9,700 ÷ 12 = $808.33

59. ($100)(.90) = $90. Then, ($90)(.98) = $88.20

60. 1,250 − (1,250)(.18) = $1,025

61. $30.45/$870 = 3.5%. Then, 3.5% of $1,500 = $52.50

62. (.035)(60/360) = .00583̄ = discount for 60 days.
    The value of the note = (1 − .00583̄)($3500) = $3,479.58.

63. W = 5.5(20+6) = (5.5)(26) = 143

64. x/80 = 40/100. Solving, x = 32. Note that AD:AC = DE:BC

65. When folded, each new side is √49 = 7

EXAMINATION SECTION
TEST 1

DIRECTIONS: Each question or incomplete statement is followed by several suggested answers or completions. Select the one that BEST answers the question or completes the statement. *PRINT THE LETTER OF THE CORRECT ANSWER IN THE SPACE AT THE RIGHT.*

1. John is 1/6 of his father's age. In 20 years, he will be 1/2 of his father's age at that time. How old is the father?

    A. 24 B. 30 C. 36 D. 42 E. 48

2. (.7/.07)(49/100) = 4 + x x =

    A. 4.9 B. .09 C. .9 D. 3.1 E. 3.95

3. Which is the largest?

    A. 23/25 B. 27/30 C. 15/16 D. 14/15 E. 7/8

4. Clyde received a 10% raise in each of the last two years. His present salary is $43,560. What was his starting salary?

    A. $36,000 B. $38,000 C. $40,000 D. $42,700 E. $52,708

5. At a convention of dentists, 1,000 dentists are from the east coast. One hundred dentists are women; 60 of the women are not from the east coast. How many male dentists are from the east coast?

    A. 900 B. 850 C. 800 D. 960 E. 940

6. 1/3 of 1/4 is what percent of 5/12?

    A. .2 B. 5 C. 12 D. 20 E. 500

7. Which line is parallel to the y axis?

    A. x = 4y
    B. x = 2/y⁰
    C. x = y + 6
    D. xy = 2
    E. xy = 2 + 4y⁻¹

8. The five tires that come with Mary's new car were rotated frequently so that each tire was used for exactly the same amount of time as the others. They were replaced when the odometer read 24,000 miles. How many miles had each been driven?

    A. 18,000 miles
    B. 30,000 miles
    C. 20,000 miles
    D. 24,000 miles
    E. 19,200 miles

9. $\dfrac{-\binom{7646}{x}}{4---}$ What is the smallest number x could be?

    A. 2647 B. 4000 C. 3000 D. 646 E. 3646

123

10. A bug sits at the edge of a 12 inch (diameter) phonograph record playing at 33 1/3 r.p.m. Approximately how fast (in feet/minute) is the bug moving?

    A. 3 B. 33 C. 50 D. 100 E. 396

11. An object floats if it weighs less than an equal volume of water. One cc of water weighs 1 gram. Each of the following objects weighs 2 kilograms.
    Which ones float? (All dimensions in cm.)

    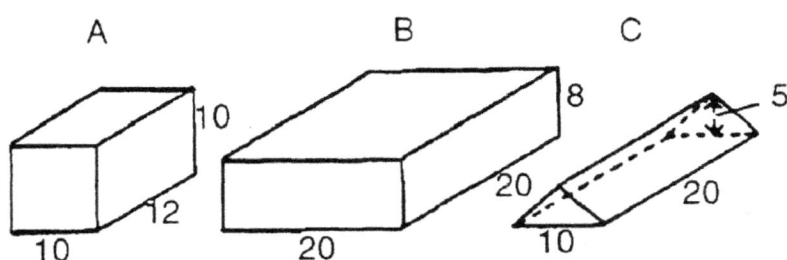

    A. A only B. B only C. C only D. B & C E. A & B

12. .04 is 25% of

    A. 0.01 B. 0.16 C. 0.1 D. 1.0 E. 1.6

13. $x^2 + 3x + 2 = 2$, $x < 0$.
    x =

    A. $\frac{3-\sqrt{8}}{2}$ B. -1 C. -2 D. -3 E. -4

14. if 3x/4y = 1/8, then 4x/3y =

    A. 1/6 B. 1/3 C. 2/3 D. 24 E. 2/9

15. .3% of 25% equals

    A. 7.5 B. .75 C. .075 D. .0075 E. .00075

16. Arrange from least to greatest:

    I. .07   II. $\sqrt{.49}$ III. .075   IV. $(.835)^2$

    The CORRECT answer is:

    A. I, III, IV, II
    B. III, I, IV, II
    C. IV, I, II, III
    D. I, III, II, IV
    E. IV, II, III, I

17. A television set is priced at $490.00. The installment payment contract requires 20% of the price as a down-payment, plus installments of $47.75 per month over a period of 10 months to pay for the set, including interest charges.
    What is the total amount of interest charged?

    A. $83.00 B. $83.50 C. $85.50 D. $85.75 E. $125.50

18. A florist bought some plants for $150. He sold enough at 75 cents to meet the cost and had 100 plants left. How many were originally purchased by the florist?

    A. 150   B. 250   C. 300   D. 350   E. 400

19. If $3x + y = 5$ and $5x + y = 6$, then $y =$

    A. 2/7   B. .5   C. 1   D. 2   E. 3.5

20. A purse contains $3.20 in dimes and quarters. There are 3 less dimes than quarters. How many dimes are there?

    A. 7   B. 10   C. 13   D. 16   E. 20

21. A lawn fertilizer is most effective if 25 pounds is spread over 10,000 square feet. A weed killer must be mixed with the fertilizer but only 3 pounds should be used on every 15,000 square feet. What should the ratio be between the fertilizer and the weed killer when mixed?

    A. 12.5 to 1   B. 3 to 2
    C. 8.33 to 1   D. 5.5 to 1
    E. 25 to 3

22. If 1 yard = .9 meters, then 1.5 meters = how many yards?

    A. 1.65   B. 1.80   C. 1.60   D. 1.67   E. 1.35

23. ( ) is to 40 as x/5 is to ( ).

    A. 4; x/50   B. 10; 40x   C. 8; x   D. 10; 8x   E. 5; x/40

24. What is the approximate value of $\sqrt{360}$?

    A. 60   B. 18   C. 6   D. 16   E. 19

25. An auto travels at an average of 45 mi/hr for 1 hour and then an average of 60 mi/hr for the next half hour. What is the average speed for the entire time period in miles/hr.?

    A. 47.5   B. 50   C. 52.5   D. 55   E. 62.5

KEY (CORRECT ANSWERS)

1.	B	11.	B
2.	C	12.	B
3.	C	13.	D
4.	A	14.	E
5.	D	15.	E
6.	D	16.	A
7.	B	17.	C
8.	E	18.	C
9.	A	19.	E
10.	D	20.	A

21.	A
22.	D
23.	C
24.	E
25.	B

5 (#1)

SOLUTIONS TO PROBLEMS

1. Let the father's current age = x and John's current age = 1/6 x. In 20 years, their ages will be x + 20 and 1/6 x + 20. Then, 1/6 x + 20 = 1/2(x+20), which becomes 1/6 x + 20 = 1/2 x + 10. Solving, x = 30.

2. The left side of this equation becomes (10)(.49) = 4.9 Now, 4.9 = 4 + x. Solving, x = .9

3. Converting each fraction into a decimal equivalent, we get: .92, .9, .9375, .93, and .875, respectively. The largest is .9375 corresponding to 15/16.

4. Let x = initial salary. With the first 10% raise, his salary is 1.10x. The second 10% raise will bring his salary to (1.10x)(1.10) = 1.21x. Now, 1.21x = $43,560. Solving, x = $36,000

5. The number of female dentists from the east coast is 100 - 60 = 40. Thus, the number of male dentists from the east coast must be 1000 - 40 = 960.

6. 1/3 of 1/4 means (1/3)(1/4) = 1/12. Then, $\frac{1}{12} \div \frac{5}{12} = \frac{1}{5}$, and $\frac{1}{5}$ = 20%

7. Any line parallel to the y-axis has no slope, and so must be of the form x = c (c is a constant). $x = 2/y^0$ can be written as x = 2/1 or x = 2.

8. Since only 4 tires are used at the same time, each of the 5 tires will be used 4/5 or 80% of the elapsed time before replacement. (24,000)(.80) = 19,200.

9. To find the minimum x, we need to find the maximum for the answer (since this is a subtraction). The maximum answer upon subtracting is 4999. Solving, 7646 - x = 4999, we get x = 2647.

10. The circumference = (π)(1 foot) = 3.14 feet (approximately) 33 1/3 revolutions = (33 1/3)(3.14) = 104 2/3 feet, which is the rate per minute.

11. 2 kilograms = 2000 grams. The only object(s) which float must correspond to more than 2000 cc. Object A has a volume of only 1200 cc. Object B has a volume of 3200 cc. Object C has a volume of only (1/2)(10)(5)(20) = 500 cc. Object B will float since 3200 cc. of water weighs 3200 grams and 2000 < 3200. Objects A and C will not float.

12. Solve .04 = .25x to get x = .16.

13. Rewrite the equation as $x^2 + 3x = 0$. Then, x(x+3) = 0. The two answers are x = 0 and x = -3. With the restriction x < 0, we have x = -3.

14. 3x/4y = 1/8. Dividing both sides by 3/4, we get x/y =1/6. Now, multiply the entire equation x/y = 1/6 by 4/3 to get 4x/3y = (1/6)(4/3) = 2/9

15. .3% of 25% becomes (.003)(.25) = .00075

16. The equivalent decimals are .07, .7, .075, and .697225. Arranging from least to greatest: .07, .075, .697225, and .7, which correspond to I, III, IV, and II.

17. The actual payments are (.20)($490) + (10)($47.75) = $575.50 Interest amount = $575.50 - $490 = $85.50

18. The number of plants he sold = $150 ÷ $0.75 = 200.
    Since he had 100 plants left, he originally purchased 200 + 100 = 300 plants.

19. Subtract the first equation from the second to get $2x = 1$. So, $x = .5$. Substitute this x value in either equation. Choosing the first equation, $(3)(.5) + y = 5$. Then, $y = 3.5$

20. Let x = number of dimes, x + 3 = number of quarters.
    Then, $.10x + .25(x+3) = 3.20$. Simplifying, $.35x + .75 = 3.20$. Finally, $x = 7$

21. For the weed killer, since 3 pounds should be used on 15,000 square feet, this translates into 2 pounds per 10,000 square feet. The ratio on the 10,000 square feet of lawn for fertilizer to weed killer is 25 to 2. This reduces to 12.5 to 1.

22. 1.5 meters = 1.5 ÷ .9 = 1.67 yards

23. Substituting choice C, 8 to 40 = 1/5 and x/5 to x = 1/5

24. $18^2 = 324$ and $19^2 = 361$. Thus, $\sqrt{360} \approx 19$

25. Total miles = $45 + (1/2)(60) = 75$. Total time = $1 + 1/2 = 1\ 1/2$ hours
    Average speed = $75 \div 1\ 1/2 = 50$ mi/hr.

TEST 2

DIRECTIONS: Each question or incomplete statement is followed by several suggested answers or completions. Select the one that BEST answers the question or completes the statement. *PRINT THE LETTER OF THE CORRECT ANSWER IN THE SPACE AT THE RIGHT.*

1. 1/3 of 15 = 15% of
   A. 3/4   B. 45   C. 75   D. 5   E. 33 1/3

   1.____

2. A tree in an apartment building courtyard died, and the cost of cutting down the tree is $350.00. The city will share the cost with the landlord on a 2 to 3 ratio, the landlord paying the larger part. How much will the landlord have to pay?

   A. $233.00   B. $175.00
   C. $117.00   D. $150.00
   E. $210.00

   2.____

3. $\frac{1}{2} + \frac{4}{2x-1} = 6$. x =
   A. - 1/2   B. 13/22   C. 19/22   D. - 1/4   E. - 15/22

   3.____

4. The capacity of a car's cooling system if 17 quarts. 1 3/4 gallons of antifreeze plus 1 pint of rust inhibitor are required to drop the freezing point to -18°. How much water is required to fill the system to capacity?

   A. 21 pints   B. 9 pints
   C. 19 pints   D. 10 quarts
   E. 18 pints

   4.____

5. If 1 inch = 2.54 cm., 3/4 cm. = how many inches?
   A. 1.9   B. 3.39   C. .75   D. .19   E. .3

   5.____

6. A box has the shape of a rectangular solid, with a base measuring 16 inches by 10 inches and a height of 8 inches. What is the approximate length of the sides of a cubic container having the same volume?

   A. 9.75 inches   B. 10.00 inches
   C. 10.85 inches   D. 12.65 inches
   E. 13.15 inches

   6.____

7. What is a valid formula for the line plotted on the graph?
   A. x = y
   B. x = 10/y
   C. x = 10 - y
   D. x = y/10
   E. x = y + 10

   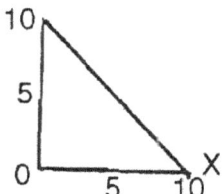

   7.____

8. In the fraction x/y, when 1 is added to the numerator, the fraction equals 1/3. When 3 is added to the denominator of x/y, the fraction equals 1/6. What is x/y?

   A. 2/6   B. 2/3   C. 2/9   D. 6/17   E. 2/12

   8.____

9. What is the *approximate* value of $\frac{(.03)^2(\sqrt{.25} + 3.5)}{.12}$?

   A. .03   B. .36   C. .003   D. 3.0   E. .0036

10. A woman is now three times as old as her son. In four years, the son will be one-half as old as the woman is now. How old is the woman now?

    A. 24   B. 28   C. 30   D. 21   E. 33

11. 1/5 of 27 = 25% of

    A. 21 3/5   B. 5.4   C. 1.35   D. 105/5   E. 21.5

12. A rancher had 70 head of cattle. A buyer made four purchases of cattle from the rancher. The rancher now has eighteen cattle remaining. On the average, how many cattle exchanged hands at EACH purchase?

    A. 10.5   B. 13   C. 15   D. 20   E. 52

13. $\sqrt{16 + x} = 4 + 2$ x =

    A. 36   B. 4   C. -10   D. 20   E. 2

14. If 10 cc of 20% acid is mixed with 20 cc of 40% acid, the percentage of acid in the resulting solution is

    A. 50   B. 30   C. 33 1/3   D. 35   E. 60

15. 5/6 + 5/9 - 2/3 + x = a whole number. Then x = ?

    A. 5/18   B. 13/16   C. 17/18   D. 18/13   E. 2/9

16. A piece of lumber is 63 inches long. It is to be cut in three pieces. Two pieces are to be of equal length, while the third piece is to be 9 inches longer than each of the other two pieces. How long will the longer piece of lumber be?

    A. 54 inches   B. 36 inches
    C. 30 inches   D. 27 inches
    E. 18 inches

17. The sun shining on a tree casts a shadow 45 feet long. A boy five feet tall standing near the tree has a 2 foot 10 inch shadow. How tall is the tree?

    A. 54 feet   B. 22.5 feet
    C. 37.5 feet   D. 79.4 feet
    E. 18 feet

18. x/95 = 7.5% x =

    A. 12.7   B. 7.1   C. 8.0   D. 1.26   E. 713

19. A street light shining on a signpost casts a shadow 6 feet long. A child 5 feet tall standing near the signpost casts a shadow 2 feet 3 inches long. How tall is the signpost?

    A. 13.3 feet   B. 6.6 feet
    C. 12 feet   D. 20 feet
    E. 15.3 feet

20. $\dfrac{(-2)^{15}}{(-2)^{12}} = ?$

   A. -4   B. +4   C. -8   D. +8   E. -16

21. Five consecutive whole numbers have a sum of 50. What is the second of the five numbers?

   A. 5   B. 7   C. 9   D. 10   E. 11

22. If z = 35% of w, and y = 15% of z, then y = _____% of w.

   A. 2.33   B. 42.9   C. 5.25   D. 2.25   E. 4.3

23. If (y + 2)x = 1/4, y =

   A. 1/4 - 2x
   B. 1/4x - 2
   C. 1/4x + 8
   D. x/4 - 2
   E. 1 - 8x/4

24. A set of drill bits are being sold for $200.00. The bits cost the dealer $160.00, plus a $20.00 shipping fee. What percent of the selling price will be profit for the dealer?

   A. 7%   B. 10%   C. 11%   D. 21%   E. 30%

25. Let A be the area of a circle whose diameter is 8. Which of the following numbers is closest to A?

   A. 50   B. 70   C. 100   D. 120   E. 200

KEY (CORRECT ANSWERS)

1.	E	11.	A
2.	E	12.	B
3.	C	13.	D
4.	C	14.	C
5.	E	15.	A
6.	C	16.	D
7.	C	17.	D
8.	C	18.	B
9.	A	19.	A
10.	A	20.	C

21. C
22. C
23. B
24. B
25. A

SOLUTIONS TO PROBLEMS

1. 1/3 of 15 = 5. Then, 5 ÷ .15 = 33 1/3

2. Let 2x = city's cost and 3x = landlord's cost. 2x + 3x = $350 Solving, x = $70. Then, landlord's cost is (3)($70) = $210

3. Multiplying the equation by (2)(2x-1), we get (1)(2x-1) + (4)(2) = (6)(2)(2x-1). Simplifying, 2x - 1 + 8 = 24x - 12.
   This reduces further to 19 = 22x. So, x = 19/22

4. 1 3/4 gallons = (1 3/4)(4) = 7 quarts = 14 pints of antifreeze.
   The capacity of the cooling system = 17 quarts = 34 pints. Since 1 pint of rust inhibitor is needed, the amount of water required is 34 - 14 - 1 = 19 pints.

5. 3/4 cm = 3/4 ÷ 2.54 = .295 or about .3 inches

6. The volume of the box = (16)(10)(8) = 1280 cubic inches. If a cubic container has a volume of 1280 cubic inches, each side must be $\sqrt[3]{1280} \approx 10.85$ inches.
   (Actually, the answer is slightly closer to 10.86)

7. Since the coordinates of the two given points are (10,0) and (0,10), the slope of the line is (10-0) ÷ (0-10) = -1. Y = -1x + B, where B is the y-intercept. Now, B = 10 since (0,10) lies on this line. Y = -1x + 10 is the equation and this can be written as x = 10 - y.

8. From the given information, (x+1)/y = 1/3 and x/(y+3) = 1/6 Rewriting, we have y = 3x + 3 and y = 6x - 3. Adding these equations, 2y = 9x. Thus, x/y = 2/9.

9. $(.03)^2$ = .0009. ($\sqrt{.25}$ + 3.5) = 4.0. The answer becomes (.0009)(4)/.12 = .03. (Change the word *approximate* to *exact*.)

10. Let x = woman's age, 1/3x = son's age. Then, 1/3 x + 4 = 1/2 x.
    This reduces to 1/6 x = 4, so x = 24.

11. 1/5 of 27 = (.2)(27) = 5.4. Then, 5.4 ÷ .25 = 21.6 = 21 3/5

12. 70 - 18 = 52. Then, 52 ÷ 4 = 13.

13. $\sqrt{16+x}$ = 6. Square both sides to get 16 + x = 36. Then, x = 20

14. The amount of acid in the resulting solution is (.20)(10) + (.40)(20) = 10 cc. The solution is 10 + 20 = 30 cc. Percentage of acid is (10/30)(100) = 33 1/3

15. 5/6 + 5/9 - 2/3 = (15 + 10 - 12)/18 = 13/18. Since choice A is 5/18, 13/18 + 5/18 = 18/18 = 1, which is a whole number.

16. Let x = length of each shorter piece and x + 9 = length of the longer piece. x + x + x + 9 = 63. Solving, x = 18. So, the longer piece must be 27 inches.

17. The ratio of the boy's height to his shadow is 60 inches to 34 inches = 30 to 17 (reduced). Let x = height of the tree. Then, x/45 = 30/17. Solving, x ≈ 79.4 feet

5 (#2)

18. x/95 = .075. x = (.075)(95) = 7.125 or about 7.1   18._____

19. The ratio of the child's height to his shadow is 60 inches to 27 inches = 20 to 9 (reduced). 19._____
    Let x = height of the signpost. Then, x/6 = 20/9. Solving, x - 13.33 or about 13.3 feet.

20. In division, we subtract exponents to get $(-2)^3$ = -8. Of course, the base must remain the   20._____
    same.

21. Let x, x+1, x+2, x+3, x+4 represent the numbers. Then, x + x+1 + x+2 + x+3 + x+4 = 50. 21._____
    Solving, x = 8. The second number must be 9.

22. y = .15z = (.15)(.35)w = .0525w. Thus, y is 5.25% of w.   22._____

23. (y+2)(x) = 1/4. Dividing both sides by x, we get y + 2 = 1/4x. Finally, y = 1/4x - 2   23._____

24. The dealer's total cost is $180 and his profit is $20. The percent profit on the selling price 24._____
    is (20/200)(100) = 10%.

25. A=$(\pi)(4)^2$ = 16π = 50.265 or about 50. Note that the formula is Area = (π) (radius)^2. 25._____

ARITHMETICAL REASONING
EXAMINATION SECTION
TEST 1

DIRECTIONS: Each question or incomplete statement is followed by several suggested answers or completions. Select the one that BEST answers the question or completes the statement. *PRINT THE LETTER OF THE CORRECT ANSWER IN THE SPACE AT THE RIGHT.*

Questions 1-4.

DIRECTIONS: In answering questions 1-4, assume that you are working in a medical facility and are responsible for maintaining inventory and stock.

1. The following quantities of disposable syringes were used during the first six weeks of the year: 840, 756, 772, 794, 723, and 789.
   If the cost of a disposable syringe is seventy cents, the average weekly cost for disposable syringes is MOST NEARLY

   A. $550   B. $780   C. $850   D. $3,270

2. Four pieces of glass tubing measuring 4 feet 3 inches, 6 feet 8 inches, 7 feet 2 inches, and 7 feet 6 inches are to be cut into 5-inch pieces.
   The TOTAL number of 5-inch pieces that can be cut from the four pieces is

   A. 60   B. 61   C. 62   D. 63

3. Assume that a 55-gallon drum of disinfectant is to be distributed equally among eight work stations.
   The amount of disinfectant that each work station should receive is

   A. 7.5 gallons   B. 27.5 pints
   C. 55 pints   D. 55 quarts

4. On June 30, an inventory indicated that there were 13 dozen petri dishes in the stockroom. During the next four weeks in July, the following quantities of petri dishes were given out by the stockroom: 23, 56, 37, and 31. On August 1, no petri dishes were given out, but 9 dozen were delivered to the stockroom.
   The number of petri dishes in the stockroom AFTER delivery on August 1 is

   A. 18   B. 108   C. 110   D. 117

5. A table of composition of foods lists the protein value of a 100 gram portion of hamburger at 22 grams. The protein value of a 45 gram portion of hamburger is, therefore, _____ grams.

   A. 5   B. 9.9   C. 11.3   D. 12.4

6. To cover a room 15' x 18' with wall-to-wall carpeting requires _____ square yards.

   A. 25   B. 30   C. 35   D. 90

7. Assume that you are in a hospital whose x-ray department is open from 8 A.M. to 12 Noon and from 1 P.M. to 6 P.M. You have assigned one of your technicians to schedule all the x-ray appointments for the clinic cases. Your instructions to him are not to make more than 12 appointments per half hour in the morning session and not more 15 per hour for the afternoon session.
   The GREATEST number of patients he can schedule in the entire day will be
   A. 75   B. 96   C. 123   D. 171

8. 1,000,000 may be represented as
   A. 10^3 B. 10^5 C. 10^6 D. 10^{10}

9. 35° Centigrade equals
   A. 70° F   B. 95° F   C. 100° F   D. 120° F

10. $10^3 \times 10^4$ equals
    A. 10^7 B. 10^{12} C. 100^7 D. 100^{12}

11. If a mixture is made up of one part Substance A, 3 parts Substance B, and 12 parts Substance C, the proportion of Substance A in the mixture is
    A. 4%   B. 6 1/4%   C. 16%   D. 62 1/2%

12. If 5 grams of a chemical are enough to perform a certain laboratory test 9 times, the quantity of the chemical needed to perform this test 1,350 times would be _____ grams.
    A. 30   B. 150   C. 270   D. 750

13. If it takes 7 grams of a certain substance to make 5 liters of a solution, the quantity of the substance needed to make 4 liters of the solution is _____ grams.
    A. 2.85   B. 4.70   C. 5.60   D. 8.75

14. If it takes 3 grams of Substance A and 7 grams of Substance B to make 4 liters of a solution, how many grams of Substances A and B does it take to make 5 liters of the solution?
    _____ of Substance A and _____ of Substance B.
    A. 3.35; 6.65   B. 3.50; 7.50
    C. 3.75; 8.75   D. 4; 7

15. A certain type of laboratory test can be performed by a laboratory technician in 20 minutes.
    Three laboratory technicians can perform 243 such tests in _____ hours.
    A. 16   B. 20   C. 27   D. 81

16. Pairs of shatterproof plastic safety glasses cost $38.00 each, but an 8% discount is given on orders of six pairs or more. Pairs of straight blade dissecting scissors cost $144 a dozen with a 12% discount on orders of two dozen or more.
    The TOTAL cost of eight pairs of safety glasses and 30 pairs of dissecting scissors is MOST NEARLY
    A. $596.50   B. $621.00   C. $664.00   D. $731.50

17. On July 1, your laboratory has 280 usable 20-gauge needles on hand. On August 1, 15% of these needles have been lost or damaged beyond repair. On August 15, a new shipment of 50 needles is received by the laboratory, but 10% of these arrive damaged and are returned to the seller.
    At this point, the number of usable 20-gauge needles on hand would be

    A. 238   B. 283   C. 288   D. 325

17._____

18. A certain laboratory procedure can be completed by a laboratory technician in 15 minutes.
    If your lab is assigned 30 such tests, and they must be completed within 3 hours, the MINIMUM number of technicians that would have to be assigned to this task is

    A. 2   B. 3   C. 4   D. 5

18._____

19. A patient's hospital bill is $24,600. The patient has three different medical insurance plans, each of which will make partial payment toward his bill. One plan will pay $6,500 of the patient's bill, another will pay $7,300 of the bill, and the third will pay $8,832 of the bill. The percentage of the bill that the patient's three insurance plans combined do NOT pay for is

    A. 5%   B. 8%   C. 10%   D. 20%

19._____

20. A patient has stayed at a hospital for which the all-inclusive daily rate is $205.00. The patient was hospitalized for 27 days. The patient is covered by a private insurance plan that will pay the hospital 2/3 of the patient's total hospital bill.
    The one of the following that MOST NEARLY indicates how much of the patient's hospital bill would NOT be covered by this insurance plan is

    A. $1,845   B. $2,078   C. $3,690   D. $3,156

20._____

21. A hospital charges a flat daily rate for all hospital services. In February 2000, the hospital charged a patient $2,772 for 14 days of hospitalization. In April 2002, the same patient was charged for 16 days of hospitalization at the same hospital.
    If the daily rate charged by the hospital increased by $7 between the patient's 2000 hospitalization and his 2002 hospitalization, the total amount that the patient must pay for the 2002 hospitalization is

    A. $3,296   B. $3,280   C. $3,264   D. $3,248

21._____

22. A hospital insurance plan that previously covered 3/5 of the total hospital charges for its subscribers has recently been improved, and coverage for total hospital charges has been increased by 25% of the previous rate. A subscriber to this plan has just completed a hospital stay and has received a bill for total hospital charges of $6,200.
    Assuming that the hospital stay is covered by the recently improved plan, the one of the following that MOST NEARLY indicates how much the plan now provides the patient toward the payment of the hospital bill is

    A. $1,550   B. $3,720   C. $4,650   D. $5,270

22._____

4 (#1)

Questions 23-25.

DIRECTIONS: Questions 23 through 25 are to be answered on the basis of the following situation.

You have been asked to keep records of the time spent with each patient by the doctors in the clinic where you are assigned. Your notes show that Dr. Jones spent the following amount of time with each patient he examined on a certain day: Patient A - 14 minutes, Patient B - 13 minutes, Patient C - 34 minutes, Patient D - 48 minutes, Patient E - 26 minutes, Patient F - 20 minutes, Patient G - 25 minutes.

23. The average number of minutes spent by Dr. Jones with each patient is MOST NEARLY   23.___

    A. 20   B. 25   C. 30   D. 35

24. If Dr. Jones is to take care of the seven patients mentioned above at one session, the   24.___
    number of hours he will have to remain at the clinic is MOST NEARLY _____ hour(s).

    A. 1   B. 2   C. 3   D. 4

25. The one of the following groups of patients that required the LEAST time to examine is   25.___
    Patients _____ and _____.

    A. A, C; E   B. B, D; F   C. C, E; G   D. A, D; G

KEY (CORRECT ANSWERS)

1. A
2. B
3. C
4. D
5. B

6. B
7. D
8. C
9. B
10. A

11. B
12. D
13. C
14. C
15. C

16. A
17. B
18. B
19. B
20. A

21. B
22. C
23. B
24. C
25. A

SOLUTIONS TO PROBLEMS

1. $(840+756+772+794+723+789) \div 6 = 779$. Then, $(779)(.70) = \$545.30 \approx \$550$

2. $4'3" + 6'8" + 7'2" + 7'6" = 25'7" = 307"$. Then, $307 \div 5 = 61.4$, so 61 5-inch pieces exist.

3. $55 \div 8 = 6.875$ gallons = 55 pints

4. $(13)(12) - 23 - 56 - 37 - 31 + (9)(12) = 117$ dishes

5. Let x = protein value. Then, Solving, x = 9.9 grams

6. $(15')(18') = 270$ sq.ft. = 30 sq.yds.

7. Maximum number of appointments = $(12)(8) + (15)(5) = 171$

8. $1,000,000 = 10^6$

9. $F = 9/5\,C + 32$. If $C = 35$, $F = (9/5)(35) + 32 = 95$

10. $10^3 \times 10^4 = 10^7$. When multiplying with like bases, add the exponents.

11. $\dfrac{1}{1+3+2} = \dfrac{1}{16} = 6\dfrac{1}{4}\%$

12. Let x = grams needed. Then, $5/9 = x/1350$. Solving, x = 750

13. Let x = grams needed. Then, $7/5 = x/4$ Solving, x = 5.6

14. Let x = grams of A needed and y = grams of B needed. Then, $3/4 = x/5$ and $7/4 = y/5$ Solving, x = 3.75, y = 8.75

15. The test requires 1/3 technician-hrs. Now, $(243)(1/3) = 81$ technician-hrs., and $81 \div 3 = 27$ hours

16. $(8)(\$38.00)(.92) + (2\,1/2)(\$144)(.88) = \$596.48 \approx \$596.50$

17. $280 - (.15)(280) + 50 - (.10)(50) = 283$ needles on hand

18. The test requires 1/4 technician-hrs., so 30 tests require 7 1/2 technician-hrs. Since 3 hrs. is the time limit for these 30 tests, $7\,1/2 \div 3 = 2.5$ or 3 technicians at a minimum are needed.

19. $\$24,600 - (\$6500+\$7300+\$8832) = \$1968$, and $1968/24,600 = 8\%$

20. Amount not covered = $(1/3)(\$205)(27) = \$1845$

21. Daily rate for 2000 = $\$2772 \div 14 = \$198$, so for 2002 the daily rate = $\$205$. Finally, $(\$205)(16) = \$3280$

22. The new plan covers $(.60)(1.25) = .75$ or 75% of the bill. Then, $(.75)(\$6200) = \$4650$

23. (14+13+34+48+26+20+25) ÷ 7 ≈ 26 min., closest to 25 min.

24. 180 min. = 3 hours

25. Patients A, C, E: 74 min.; patients B, D, F: 81 min.; patients C, E, G: 85 min.; patients A, D, G: 87 min. So, the 1st group requires the least time.

TEST 2

DIRECTIONS: Each question or incomplete statement is followed by several suggested answers or completions. Select the one that BEST answers the question or completes the statement. *PRINT THE LETTER OF THE CORRECT ANSWER IN THE SPACE AT THE RIGHT.*

1. A stack of cartons containing pesticides is 10 cartons long, 9 cartons wide, and 5 cartons high.
   The number of cartons in the stack is

   A. 24   B. 55   C. 95   D. 450

   1.____

2. Assume that you have bags of corn meal, each of the same weight. The total weight of 25 bags is 125 pounds.
   How many of these bags would it take to make a TOTAL weight of 50 pounds?

   A. 2   B. 5   C. 6   D. 10

   2.____

3. You are working in the sub-basement of a project building, and the foreman tells you to get two boards from the maintenance shop to stand on. One of the boards is 5 yards long, and the other 3 1/2 feet long.
   The TOTAL length, in feet, of the two boards is

   A. 8 1/2   B. 9 1/2   C. 17 1/2   D. 18 1/2

   3.____

4. Three hundred plastic bags of rat-mix, each bag weighing four ounces, are packed in a carton. The carton weighed one pound before the rat-mix was packed in it.
   The TOTAL weight of the filled carton is _____ pounds.

   A. 37 1/2   B. 38 1/2   C. 75   D. 76

   4.____

5. Of 180 families that relocated in a given month, 1/5 moved into Finder's Fee apartments, 1/4 moved into tenant-found apartments, 1/3 moved into public housing, and the rest moved out of the city.
   How many moved out of the city?

   A. 36   B. 39   C. 45   D. 60

   5.____

6. If a space treatment device covers 1,000 cubic feet in six seconds, how long should it run in order to treat a room that is 30 feet long, 20 feet wide, and 15 feet high?

   A. 18 seconds   B. 54 seconds
   C. 1 minute 24 seconds   D. 1 minute 48 seconds

   6.____

7. If you have to prepare five gallons of 0.5 Diazinon emulsion using water and 20% Diazinon emulsifiable concentrate, what is the amount of concentrate that is necessary? _____ ounces.

   A. 1.6   B. 3.2   C. 16.0   D. 64.0

   7.____

8. Suppose you have 15 5/6 ounces of a certain chemical on hand.
   If you later receive shipments of 6 1/2 ounces and 8 3/4 ounces of this chemical, the TOTAL number of ounces you should then have on hand is

   A. 29 7/8   B. 30 5/6   C. 31 1/12   D. 31 3/4

   8.____

9. You are told to prepare 60 pounds of 2% pyrethrum dust using talc and 5% pyrethrum dust concentrate.
   What is the amount of concentrate that is required in the mixture?
   _____ pounds.

   A. 24 B. 28 C. 30 1/2 D. 36

10. In the pest control shop of a certain housing development, there is a supply of 4 one-gallon containers of insecticide. This week, the exterminator will use up five quarts of this insecticide in his work, and for each week thereafter he will use up five quarts. Deliveries are made on the first day of the week.
    Next week, and each week thereafter, the shop will get a delivery of one gallon of insecticide. The exterminator will need an additional supply of insecticide by the end of the _____ week.

    A. 4th B. 12th C. 24th D. 29th

11. There are 22 boxes of rat mix in a certain pest control shop.
    If each box contains 7 1/2 pounds of rat mix, the TOTAL amount of rat mix in the shop is _____ pounds.

    A. 165 B. 172 1/2 C. 180 D. 182 1/2

12. A pest control shop has a supply of 26 one-gallon cans of insecticide.
    If the exterminator works 5 days a week and uses 32 ounces of the liquid a day, the number of work weeks this supply of insecticide will last is MOST NEARLY

    A. 10 B. 20 C. 28 D. 32

13. A certain supplier packs two dozen mousetraps to a box. If the exterminator gets a delivery of 20 boxes and finds that two of these boxes are half-full, the TOTAL number of traps the exterminator received from this supplier is

    A. 408 B. 432 C. 456 D. 480

14. Assume that a truck which contains a shipment of pesticides is parked outside your exterminating shop. You are able to unload the truck in one hour.
    How long would it take four exterminators, starting at the same time and working at the same rate as you, to unload four trucks similar to the one you unloaded?

    A. 15 minutes B. 1 hour C. 2 hours D. 4 hours

15. A certain building in a housing development has 142 apartments. It takes one exterminator an average of six minutes to treat one apartment.
    At that rate, approximately how long should it take him to treat all 142 apartments?
    _____ hours.

    A. 2 B. 14 C. 24 D. 85

16. A crate contains 3 pieces of pesticide equipment weighing 73, 84, and 47 pounds, respectively.
    If the crate is lifted by 4 exterminators, each lifting one corner of the crate, the average number of pounds, in addition to the weight of the crate, lifted by each of the exterminators is

    A. 51 B. 65 C. 71 D. 78

17. Of the following, the pair that is NOT a set of equivalents is

    A. .014%; .00014   B. 1/5%; .002   C. 1.5%; 3/200   D. 115%; .115

18. 10^{-2} is equal to

    A. 0.001   B. 0.01   C. 0.1   D. 100.0

19. $10^2 \times 10^3$ is equal to

    A. 10^5 B. 10^6 C. 100^5 D. 100^6

20. The length of two objects are in the ratio of 2:1.
    If each were 3 inches shorter, the ratio would be 3:1.
    The longer object is _____ inches.

    A. 8   B. 10   C. 12   D. 14

21. If the weight of water is 62.4 pounds per cubic foot, the weight of the water that fills a rectangular container 6 inches by 6 inches by 1 foot is _____ pounds.

    A. 7.8   B. 15.6   C. 31.2   D. 46.8

22. The formula for converting degrees Centigrade to degrees Fahrenheit is as follows:
    Fahrenheit = 9/5 of Centigrade + 32°, or
    multiply the number of degrees Centigrade by 9, divide by 5 and add 32).
    If the Centigrade thermometer reads 25°, the temperature in degrees Fahrenheit is

    A. 13   B. 45   C. 53   D. 77

23. To make a certain preparation, you have been told to mix one ounce of Liquid A and 3 ounces of Liquid B.
    If you have used 18 ounces of Liquid B in preparing a larger amount, the number of ounces of Liquid A you should use is

    A. 6   B. 15   C. 21   D. 54

24. If one inch is equal to approximately 2.5 centimeters, the number of inches in fifteen centimeters is MOST NEARLY

    A. 1.6   B. 6   C. 12.5   D. 37.5

25. You are in charge of a small lawn area of 1,850 sq. ft. You are asked to apply lime on this lawn at the rate of 40 pounds per 1,000 sq. ft.
    The number of pounds of lime you will need to cover the entire area of the lawn is MOST NEARLY _____ pounds.

    A. 74   B. 86   C. 87   D. 89

4 (#2)

KEY (CORRECT ANSWERS)

1. D
2. D
3. D
4. D
5. B

6. B
7. C
8. C
9. A
10. B

11. A
12. B
13. C
14. B
15. B

16. A
17. D
18. B
19. A
20. C

21. B
22. D
23. A
24. B
25. A

5 (#2)

SOLUTIONS TO PROBLEMS

1. (10)(9)(5) = 450 cartons

2. Let x = number of bags. Then, 25/125 = x/50 . Solving, x = 10

3. 5 yds. + 3 1/2 ft. = 15 ft. + 3 1/2 ft. = 18 1/2 ft.

4. Total weight = 1 + (300) (4/16) = 76 pounds

5. 1-1/5-1/4-1/3=13/60. Then, (180)(13/60) = 39 families

6. (30')(20')(15') = 9000 cu.ft. Let x = number of seconds, Then, $\frac{1000}{6} = \frac{9000}{X}$. Solving, x = 54

7. 1 qt. of concentrate = 16 oz.

8. 15 5/6 + 6 1/2 + 8 3/4 = 29 25/12 = 31 1/12 ounces

9. .05x = .02(60)
   x = 24

10. For the 1st week (end), there will be 16 - 5 = 11 qts. left. For each additional week, since 4 qts. are delivered but 5 qts. are used, there will be a net loss of 1 qt. Thus, at the end of 12 weeks, the supply of insecticide will be gone.

11. (22)(7 1/2) = 165 pounds

12. (26)(128) = 3328 oz., and (32)(5) = 160 oz. used each week. Finally, 3328 ÷ 160 = 20.8, closest to 20 oz.

13. (24) (18) + (12)(2) = 456 mousetraps

14. 4 trucks require 4 man-hours. Then, 4 ÷ 4=1 hour

15. (142)(6) = 852 min. = 14.2 hrs. ≈ 14 hrs.

16. Total weight = 204 lbs. Then, 204 ÷ 4 = 51 lbs.

17. 115% = 1.15, not .115

18. 10^{-2} = 1/100 = .01

19. 10^2 x 10^3 = 10^5. When multiplying with like bases, add the exponents.

20. Let x, 1/2x = lengths of the longer and shorter objects. Then, x - 3 = 3(1/2x-3). Simplifying, x - 3 = 3/2x - 9. Solving, x = 12 in.

21. (1/2')(1/2')(1') = 1/4 cu.ft. Then, (62.4)(1/4) = 15.6 pounds

22. F = (9/5)(25°) + 32° = 77°

145

23. Let x = number of ounces of liquid A. Then, 1/3 = x/18. Solving, x = 6

24. 15 cm. = $\dfrac{15}{\approx 2.5}$ or approx. 6 in.

25. (40)(1850/1000) = 74 pounds

MATHEMATICS PROBLEM SOLVING

EXAMINATION SECTION
TEST 1

DIRECTIONS: Each question or incomplete statement is followed by several sug-gested answers or completions. Select the one that BEST answers the question or completes the statement. *PRINT THE LETTER OF THE CORRECT ANSWER IN THE SPACE AT THE RIGHT.*

1. Mr. Marsh left an estate amounting to $24,000. By his will, 10% was to be given to a college, 15% to a church, and the remainder was to be divided equally among 3 nieces. How much money did *each* niece receive?

    A. $6120 B. $2000 C. $6333.33
    D. $6000 E. *None of these answers*

2. After selling one third of his apple crop, a farmer sold the remainder at the same price per bushel for $600. What was the *value* of the crop?

    A. $1000 B. $1200 C. $1800 D. $800
    E. *None of these answers*

3. A village has an assessed valuation of $2,400,000. The rate for school taxes is 80¢ per $100 valuation. If all but 2% of the taxes are collected, how many dollars remain *uncollected*?

    A. $18,816 B. $48,000 C. $384 D. $600
    E. *None of these answers*

4. When a = 2, c = 1, and d = 0, what is the value of the expression $4a + 2c^2 - 3d^2$?

    A. 7 B. 9 C. 12 D. 15
    E. *None of these answers*

5. The difference between one half of a number and one fifth of it is 561. Find the number.

    A. 168 B. 2805 C. 1870 D. 5610
    E. *None of these answers*

6. Two triangles of the same shape are *always*

    A. similar B. equilateral C. congruent
    D. symmetrical E. equal

7. Which of the following is the BEST illustration of con-gruence?

    A. A pair of shoes
    B. Two dinner plates from the same set of dishes
    C. Any two tables
    D. A can of fruit and a cylinder
    E. A slide and its projection on a screen

8. On the average, 5 oranges will give 3 cupfuls of juice. 8.____
   If 2 cupfuls make a pint, how many oranges must be used to make 3 gallons of juice?
   A. 16 B. 20 C. 80
   D. 40 E. None of the above

9. What is the difference in cost to a purchaser between an article listed at $500 9.____
   less 10% and 20% and one listed at $490 less 20%?
   A. $18 B. $42 C. $58
   D. $48 E. None of the above

10. A salesman receives a monthly salary of $80, a 2% commission on all 10.____
    monthly sales over $2,000 and an additional 1% commission on all sales over $11,000 a month.
    If his total sales for January came to $13,500, how much did he earn that month?
    A. 355 B. 365 C. 385
    D. 405 E. 415

3 (#1)

KEY (CORRECT ANSWERS)

1. CORRECT ANSWER: D ($6,000)
   Since Mr. Marsh left 10% to a college and 15% to a church, 75% of his estate was to be equally divided among the three nieces, that is, 25% each. ¼ × $24,000 = $6,000.

2. CORRECT ANSWER: E (None of the above)
   Let x = the value of the crop. 2/3x = $600, x = $900.

3. CORRECT ANSWER: C ($384)
   Divide $2,400,000 by 100 to obtain the number of hundreds. The number is 24,000. 24,000 × .80 = $19,200 (total taxes to be collected) and $19,200 × .02 = $384 (taxes uncollected).

4. CORRECT ANSWER: E (None of the above)
   $4a + 2c^2 - 3d^2$ $4 \times 2 + 2 \times 1^2 - 30 \times 0^2 = 8 + 2 - 0 = 10$

5. CORRECT ANSWER: C (1,870)
   If x = the number, then the numbers are x/2 and x/5 (given).
   ∴ x/2 − x/5 = 561 or 3x = 5,610, x = 1,870

6. CORRECT ANSWER: A (Similar)
   By definition

7. CORRECT ANSWER: B (Two dinner plates from the same set of dishes)
   By definition, congruent figures agree in size and shape. Statement B appears to answer this requirement.

8. CORRECT ANSWER: C (80)
   Table: 2 pints = 1 quart and 4 quarts = 1 gallon. Since 8 pints = 1 gallon and 2 cupfuls = 1 pint, there are 48 cupfuls in 3 gallons. Let x – the number of oranges needed to make 3 gallons of juice. Then, 5(oranges)/3(cupfuls) = x(oranges)/48(cupfuls) or 3x = 240x = 80.

9. CORRECT ANSWER: E (None of the above)
   1. $550 × .10 = $50; $500 - $50 = $450
      $450 × .20 = $90; $450 - $90 = $360
   2. $490 × .20 = $98; $490 - $98 = $392
      $392 - $360 = $32.

10. CORRECT ANSWER: A ($355)
    Basic salary: $80 a month
    .02 × $11,500 ($13,500 - $2,000) = $230
    .01 × $2,500 ($13,500 - $11,000) = $25
    ∴ $80 + $230 + $25 = $335 (total monthly earnings)

TEST 2

DIRECTIONS: Each question or incomplete statement is followed by several suggested answers or completions. Select the one that BEST answers the question or completes the statement. *PRINT THE LETTER OF THE CORRECT ANSWER IN THE SPACE AT THE RIGHT.*

1. How much longer does it take an automobile to travel one mile at 20 miles per hour than at 30 miles per hour?
   A. 1 minute
   B. 10 minutes
   C. 20 minute
   D. 40 minutes
   E. None of the above

2. A man wishes to construct a poultry house 12 feet long in which to keep 20 hens.
   If each hen requires 4 square feet of floor space, how wide should he construct the poultry house?
   A. 28 feet
   B. 80 feet
   C. 5 feet
   D. 6 feet 8 inches
   E. None of the above

3. Aluminum bronze consists of copper and aluminum, usually in the ratio of 10:1 by weight.
   If a machine made of this alloy weighs 66 pounds, how many pounds of aluminum does it contain?
   A. 660
   B. 60
   C. 6.6
   D. 59.4
   E. None of the above

4. Mr. Brown owned a house, which he rented for $600 a month. The house was assessed at $90,000. In 2005 the rate of taxation was increased from $250 to $280 per $10,000 assessed valuation.
   By what amount should the monthly rent have been RAISED to absorb the increase in that year's taxes?
   A. $72.00
   B. $22.50
   C. $30.00
   D. $210
   E. None of the above

5. A dealer bought 3 gross of pencils at $3.80 a dozen. He sold the pencils at $.50 each.
   How much was his profit per gross?
   A. $79.20
   B. $26.40
   C. $2.20
   D. $6.60
   E. None of the above

6. How many cubic yards of earth had to be removed to make an excavation 30 feet long, 21 feet wide, and 6 feet deep?
   A. 1,260
   B. 3,780
   C. 140
   D. 420
   E. None of the above

7. By what number is the area of a circle MULTIPLIED if its radius is doubled?
   A. $2\pi r$
   B. 2
   C. 3.1416
   D. 4
   E. None of the above

2 (#2)

8. The State tax rate on 2003 incomes was 2% on the first $10,000 of income subject to tax and 3% on the next $20,000 or any part thereof. By special law, the State allowed a deduction of ¼ of the tax computed on the above schedule. In 2003, $18,000 of Mr. Brown's income was subject to tax.
   What was the amount of his tax?
   A. $110
   B. $270
   C. $330
   D. $90
   E. None of the above

   8.____

9. A baseball team won w games and lost 1 game. What fractional part of its games did it win?
   A. 1/W
   B. W/1
   C. W – 1/W
   D. W + 1/W
   E. None of the above

   9.____

10. A pole is held upright by 3 guy wires, each fastened to the pole 12 feet above the ground. The other ends of these wires are fastened to stakes 16 feet from the foot of the pole.
    Find the number of feet of wire required if 2 feet are added to each guy wire for making connections.
    A. 18 feet
    B. 66 feet
    C. 90 feet
    D. 54 feet
    E. None of the above

    10.____

KEY (CORRECT ANSWERS)

1. **CORRECT ANSWER: A (1 minute)**
   1. Since the automobile travels 1 mile at 20 miles per hour, it covers 20 miles in 1 hour or 1 mile in 3 minutes (60/20).
   2. Since the automobile travels 1 mile at 30 miles per hour, it covers 30 miles in 1 hour or 1 mile in 2 minutes (60/30)
   3. ∴ it takes automobile (1) 1 minute more than automobile (2) (3 minutes – 2 minutes = 1 minute)

2. **CORRECT ANSWER: D (6 feet 8 inches)**
   Total area of poultry house = 4 sq. ft. × 2 hens = 80 sq. ft.
   Formula: length × width = area
   Since the length, 12 ft., is given, we may represent the width by w.
   ∴ 12 × w = 80, w = 6 $\frac{2}{3}$ ft. = 6 feet 8 inches

3. **CORRECT ANSWER: E (None of the above)**
   In other words, 1 lb. of every 11 pounds of aluminum bronze is aluminum
   ∴ 1/11 × 66 lbs. = 6 lbs.

4. **CORRECT ANSWER: B ($22.50)**
   First rate of taxation: $90,000 (assessment) × .25 ($250 per $10,000)
                   = $2,250 (total taxes)
   Second rate of taxation (2005): $90,000 (assessment) × .28 ($280 per $10,000)
                   = $2,520 (total taxes)
   The increase in taxes = $270 per year ($2,520 - $2,250);
   ∴ the monthly rent should have been raised $22.50 ($270/12).

5. **CORRECT ANSWER: B ($26.40)**
   Since the selling price per dozen = $6.00 (.5 × 12) and the cost = $3.80 (given) per dozen, the profit per dozen = $2.20 ($6.00 - $3.80).
   ∴ the profit per gross (= 12 doz.) = $2.20 × 12 = $26.40

6. **CORRECT ANSWER: C (140)**
   Change the feet to yards since we are to deal with cubic yards.
   Formula: Volume = length × width × depth.
   By substitution, volume = 10 yds. × 7 yds. × 2 yds. = 140 cu. yds.

7. **CORRECT ANSWER: D (4)**
   Formula: Area of a circle = π^2
   If x = radius of original circle, then 2x = radius of new circle.
   Area of original circle $\pi \times 2$; area of new circle = $\pi(2x)^2 = 4\pi x^2$
   ∴ the area of the original circle has been multiplied by 4.

4 (#2)

8. CORRECT ANSWER: C ($330
   $10,000 × .02 = $200 (2% tax on the first $10,000)
   $8,000 × .03 = $240 (3% tax on the next $20,000, in this case $18,000, or $8,000).
   Total tax computed = $440; deduction = $110 (1/4 × $440).
   ∴ $440 - $110 = $330 (Mr. Brown's tax).

9. CORRECT ANSWER: E (None of the above)
   Formula: won/played = fractional part of games won.
   Games won = w; games played = w + 1
   ∴ w/w + 1 = fraction part of games won.

10. CORRECT ANSWER: B (66 feet)
    A right triangle is formed.
    Let x = the length of each guy wire.
    ∴ $x^2 = 12^2 + 16^2$ or $x^2 = 400$; x = 20 ft.; 20 ft. + 2 ft. = total length of each guy wire for making connections = 22 ft.
    ∴ 22 ft. × 3 = 66 ft. (total amount of wire needed for all 3 guy wires).

TEST 3

DIRECTIONS: Each question or incomplete statement is followed by several suggested answers or completions. Select the one that BEST answers the question or completes the statement. *PRINT THE LETTER OF THE CORRECT ANSWER IN THE SPACE AT THE RIGHT.*

1. What is the number of feet traversed in 1 second by an automobile that is traveling 30 miles an hour?
   A. 176
   B. 2
   C. 2,640
   D. 44
   E. None of the above

2. The Jonesville Construction Company borrowed $225,000 for five years at 3 ½%.
   What was the ANNUAL charge for interest?
   A. $1,575
   B. $1,555
   C. $7,875
   D. $39,375
   E. None of the above

3. The stock that Mr. Ames bought cost him $80 a share. The par value of the stock is $100.
   If the stock pays $6 a year in dividends, what rate of interest is Mr. Ames getting on his money?
   A. 16 ⅔%
   B. 7 ½%
   C. 3%
   D. 6%
   E. None of the above

4. The figure shown at the right represents a rectangle whose dimensions are l and w, surmounted by a semicircle whose radius is r. Express the area of this figure in terms of l, w, r and π.
   A. wl + πr²/2
   B. lw + πr²
   C. lw + πr
   D. π/2-r²lw
   E. None of the above

5. If one machine can do a piece of work in 10 hours and a second machine can do the same work in 15 hours, how many hours will it take BOTH machines working simultaneously to do the work?
   A. 12 ½
   B. 25
   C. 5
   D. 6
   E. None of the above

6. A baseball diamond is a square 90 feet on a side. Find, correct to the nearest foot, the distance from third base to first base.
   A. 180 feet
   B. 135 feet
   C. 127 feet
   D. 90 feet
   E. None of the above

2 (#3)

7. A painted wooden cube whose edge is 3 inches is cut into 27 one-inch cubes. How many of these small cubes have just two painted sides?
   A. 12
   B. 18
   C. 8
   D. 9
   E. None of the above

   7._____

8. A certain lending library charges a cents for the first week that a book is loaned and b cents for each day over one week.
   Write the formula for C, the cost in cents, of taking a book for d days from this library, (d > 7).
   A. C = a + bd
   B. C = a + b(d-7)
   C. C + ad
   D. C = 7a + b(d-7)
   E. None of the above

   8._____

9. How many gallons of water must be added to 20 gallons of a 10% solution of salt and water to REDUCE it to an 8% solution?
   A. 10
   B. 2
   C. 16
   D. 4
   E. None of the above

   9._____

10. The net profit of the ABC Company dropped from 34 million dollars in 2014 to 33 million in 2015.
    What percent of decrease does this represent? (Give answer correct to the nearest tenth of a percent)
    A. 97.0
    B. 2.9
    C. 3.0
    D. 97.1
    E. None of the above

    10._____

KEY (CORRECT ANSWERS)

1. CORRECT ANSWER: D (44)
   If the auto is traveling 30 miles an hour, this means that the auto covers 30 miles in one hour, or ½ mile in one minute (30 miles = 60 min.). To convert to seconds, as the answer calls for, divide ½ by 60 sec., viz, 1/2/60 = 1/120 mile in one second.
   Then, 120/x × 5,280 ft. (= 1 mile) = 44 ft. in one second.

2. CORRECT ANSWER: C ($7,875)
   Formula: Principal × rate × time = interest $225,000 × .035 × 1 yr. = $7,875.

3. CORRECT ANSWER: B (7 ½%)
   Formula: Principal × rate = interest (or dividend). Let x = rate of interest.
   By substitution, $80 × $6 or x = 6/80, x = .075 or 7 ½%

4. CORRECT ANSWER: A (wl + $\pi r^2/2$)
   This figure represents both a rectangle and a semicircle.
   Formulas: Area of rectangle = l (length) ×w (width) or lw or wl
   Area of semicircle: $\pi r^2$2
   Area of this figure = wl + $\pi r^2/2$

5. CORRECT ANSWER: D (6)
   Formula: Time worked/Time required = Part of job completed
   Let x = number of hours it will take both machines together to do work.
   Then, x/10 = work of one machine and x/15 = work of second machine.
   We now form the equation: x/10 + x/15 = 1 (the entire job) or 15x + 10x = 150, or 25x = 150, x = 6.

6. CORRECT ANSWER: C (127 feet)
   A right triangle is formed when a line, x, is drawn from third base to first base.
   ∴ $x^2 = 90^2 + 90^2$ or $x^2 = 16,200x$,
   x = 127.2 ft. or 127 ft. (to the nearest foot).

   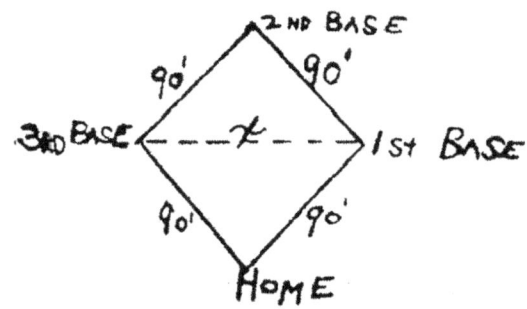

7. CORRECT ANSWER: A (12)
   By inspection

8. CORRECT ANSWER: B (C = a + b(d-7))
   a = cents charged for first week
   b = cents charged for each day over one week
   d-7 = extra days beyond the first week (given: d > 7)
   ∴ C = a + b(d-7)

4 (#3)

9. CORRECT ANSWER: E (None of the above)
Let x = number of gallons of water that must be added.
Then, 20 + x = quantity of solution after water is added.
10% × 20 gal. = 2 gal. salt in the first solution.
8% × (20+x) = amount of salt in second solution.
∴ 2 gal. (amount of salt in first solution) = .08(20+x) (amount of salt in the second solution)
or 2 = 1.60 + .08x or 8x = 40, x = 5 gal.

10. CORRECT ANSWER: B (2.9)
The drop in profit = one million dollars (34 million − 33 million)
∴ 1/34 = .0293 = 2.9% (to the nearest tenth of a percent).

TEST 4

DIRECTIONS: Each question or incomplete statement is followed by several suggested answers or completions. Select the one that BEST answers the question or completes the statement. *PRINT THE LETTER OF THE CORRECT ANSWER IN THE SPACE AT THE RIGHT.*

1. One manufacturing plant built 150 tanks in the last six months in 2005. This was an increase of 150% over the number built in the preceding six months. Find the number of tanks built in the preceding six months. 1.____
   A. 100 B. 50 C. 0
   D. 60 E. None of the above

2. What is the difference between the area of a rectangle 10 feet by 6 feet and the area of a square having the same perimeter? 2.____
   A. 165 sq.ft. B. 8 sq.ft. C. No difference
   D. 4 sq.ft. E. None of the above

3. How many cubic yards of concrete are needed to make 1,200 square concrete posts 9 inches by 6 feet? 3.____
   A. 150 B. 194,400 C. 5,400
   D. 4,050 E. None of the above

4. Find, correct to the nearest tenth of a foot, the diameter of the largest circular mirror that will pass through a doorway 7 feet high and 3 feet wide. (Neglect thickness of mirror.) 4.____
   A. 6.9 feet B. 7.0 feet C. 3.0 feet
   D. 7.6 feet E. None of the above

5. What is the GREATEST number of pictures, each 2½ inches by 3½ inches, that a photographer can print on an 8-inch by 10-inch piece of sensitized paper? 5.____
   A. 9 B. 6 C. 3
   D. 8 E. None of the above

6. The net profits of the ABC Company dropped from 35 million dollars in 2004 to 28 million in 2005.
   What percent decrease does this represent? 6.____
   A. 7% B. 20% C. 25%
   D. 80% E. None of the above

7. If 12 gallons of gas drove one car a distance of 188.4 miles and the same amount of gas took another car a distance of 202.8 miles, how much BETTER mileage per gallon has the second car than the first? 7.____
   A. 1.7 B. 5 C. 12
   D. 14.4 E. None of the above

2 (#4)

8. The length of a rectangle is 12 inches and its width is 8 inches. Let the length of the rectangle be increased by 3 inches and the width be decreased by 3 inches.
Which of the following statements is TRUE?
   A. The area of the rectangle remains the same.
   B. The area is increased by 9 square inches.
   C. The perimeter remains the same.
   D. The perimeter is increased by 6 inches.
   E. Both the perimeter and the area remain the same.

8.____

9. Approximately how many tons of coal will a bin 10 feet by 6 feet by 5 feet hold if 1 ton fills 38 cubic feet of space? (Find the answer correct to the nearest ton.)
   A. 1   B. 7   C. 3
   D. 8   E. None of the above

9.____

10. The gauge on a 10-gallon oil tank indicates that exactly 3/8 of the oil remains in the tank.
How many gallons will it require to fill the tank?
   A. 2¼   B. 3¾   C. 6½
   D. 7¼   E. None of the above

10.____

KEY (CORRECT ANSWERS)

1. CORRECT ANSWER: D (60)
   Let x = number of tanks built first half of 2005
   Let 1.5x (150%x) = increase in number of tanks built last half of 2005.
   x + 1.5x = number of tanks built last half of 2005.
   ∴ x + 1.5x = 150 or 25x = 1500, x = 60

2. CORRECT ANSWER: D (4 sq. ft.)
   Area of rectangle = length × width = 10 × 6 = 60 sq. ft.; perimeter of rectangle = 2.
   (length +width) = 2(10+6) = 32 ft.
   Perimeter of square = 32 ft. (given, same as that of rectangle)
   One side of square = 8 ft. (¼ of perimeter)
   Area of square = (side)2 = 82 = 64 sq. ft.
   ∴ 64 sq. ft. (area of square) – 60 sq. ft. (area of rectangle) = 4 sq. ft.

3. CORRECT ANSWER: A (150)
   First convert the inches and feet to yards since the answer calls for cubic yards, viz.,
   9 in. = ¼ yd. and 6 ft. = 2 yds.
   Formula: Volume (of a post) = length × width × height
   Volume (of 1200 posts) = 1200 × ¼ × ¼ × 2 = 150 cu. yds.

4. CORRECT ANSWER: D (7.6 feet)
   By drawing the diagonal (or diameter) AD, a right triangle
   is formed.
   Designate the diagonal by x.
   ∴ $x^2 = 3^2 + 7^2$ or $x^2 = 58$, x = 7.6 ft. (to the nearest
   tenth of a foot)

   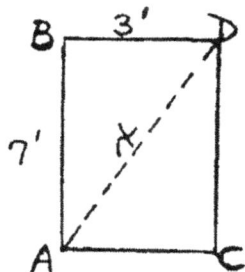

5. CORRECT ANSWER: D (8)
   This problem is solved by sketches of the only two possible ways of securing the greatest
   number of pictures, shown below.

   SKETCH 1   SKETCH 2

   8 pictures are secured when the 2½ in. side is cut along the 10 in. side of the sensitized
   paper and only 6 pictures are obtained when the 2½ in. side is cut along the 8i in. side of
   the sensitized paper.

4 (#4)

6. CORRECT ANSWER: B (20%)

$$\frac{7 \text{ (drop in net profits)(in millions of dollars)}}{35 \text{ (profit in 2004)(in millions of dollars)}} = \frac{1}{5} = 20\%$$

7. CORRECT ANSWER: E (None of the above)
The problem may be solved as follows:

Formula: $\dfrac{\text{distance}}{\text{gallons used}} = \text{mileage}$

Mileage of car 1: by substitution, $\dfrac{188.4 \text{ miles}}{12 \text{ gal}} = 15.7$ miles per gal.

Mileage of car 2: by substitution, $\dfrac{202.8 \text{ miles}}{12 \text{ gal}} = 16.9$ miles per gal.

∴ car 2 exceeds car 1 in mileage by 1.2 miles per gal.

8. CORRECT ANSWER: C (The perimeter remains the same.)
Since the area of a rectangle = length × width, the area of the original triangle = 96 sq. in. (12" × 8") and the area of the newly-formed triangle = 75 sq. in. (15" × 5").
Using this information, we find that all of the statements, except C, are false. To prove statement C is true, we use the formula: perimeter = 2 (length+width).
By substitution, we find that the perimeter of the original rectangle = 40 in. (2(12+8)), and the perimeter of the newly-formed rectangle = 40 in. (2(15+5)).

9. CORRECT ANSWER: D (8)
Formula: volume = length × width × height
By substitution, the volume of the bin = 10 × 6 × 5 = 300 cu. ft.
Let x = no. of tons of coal that the above bin will hold.
We form the proportion: 1 ton : 38 cu. ft. = x : 300 cu. ft. or 38x = 300, x = 7.8 tons or 8 tons (to the nearest ton).

10. CORRECT ANSWER: E (None of the above)
Since 3/8 of the oil is left in the tank, 5/8 more is needed to fill it.
∴ 5/8 × 10 (capacity:given) = 6¼ gal.

TEST 5

DIRECTIONS: Each question or incomplete statement is followed by several suggested answers or completions. Select the one that BEST answers the question or completes the statement. *PRINT THE LETTER OF THE CORRECT ANSWER IN THE SPACE AT THE RIGHT.*

1. A pile of steel plates is 2.75 feet high. If the plates are .375 inch thick, how many are there in the pile?
   A. 7
   B. 8
   C. 14
   D. 88
   E. None of the above

   1.____

2. At the rate of $1.50 per 6-oz. bar of chocolate, how much would a pound of chocolate cost?
   A. $3.00
   B. $3.40
   C. $3.90
   D. $4.50
   E. None of the above

   2.____

3. A man walks diagonally from one corner of a rectangular lot to the opposite corner.
   If he walks at the rate of 5 feet a second, and the lot is 50 feet by 120 feet, how many seconds will he save by walking diagonally instead of walking along the perimeter of the lot?
   A. 8
   B. 10
   C. 17
   D. 34
   E. None of the above

   3.____

4. The afternoon classes in a school begin at 1 P.M. and end at 3:52 P.M.
   There are 4 class periods with 4 minutes between classes.
   How many minutes are there in each class period?
   A. 39
   B. 40
   C. 59
   D. 60
   E. None of the above

   4.____

5. A snapshot measures $1^{7}/_{8}$" × $2\frac{1}{2}$". It is to be enlarged so that the longer dimension will be 4".
   What will be the length of the SHORTER dimension?
   A. $2^{3}/_{8}$"
   B. $2\frac{1}{2}$"
   C. 3"
   D. $3^{3}/_{8}$"
   E. None of the above

   5.____

6. The minimum temperatures at Jonesville for each day of one week were as follows: +7°, +13°, +5°, -4°, 0°, +3°.
   Find, to the nearest degree, the AVERAGE minimum temperature.
   A. 6°
   B. 2°
   C. 16°
   D. 4°
   E. None of the above

   6.____

7. If the outer diameter of an iron pipe is 14.38 inches and the inner diameter is 12.50 inches, what is the thickness of the pipe?
   A. 94"
   B. 1.88"
   C. 16.88"
   D. 26.88"
   E. None of the above

   7.____

2 (#5)

8. In the fall of 2012, a store charged $4.40 a pound for chuck steak. In February 2013, the same store had increased by 50% the price of that grade of steak. Later, the government announced a ceiling of $5.50 a pound.
What percent reduction did the store have to make in its February 2013 price in order to comply with the government ruling?
   A. 11 1/9%
   B. 16 2/3%
   C. 20%
   D. 25%
   E. None of the above

8._____

9. A certain whole number has 10 digits. If the square root of this number is taken, how many digits will there be in the integral part of the answer?
   A. 1
   B. 5
   C. 9
   D. 100
   E. None of the above

9._____

10. Four tractors working together can plow a field in 12 hours. How long will it take 6 tractors to plow a field of the same size if all tractors work at the same rate?
    A. 6 hr.
    B. 9 hr.
    C. 10 hr.
    D. 18 hr.
    E. None of the above

10._____

KEY (CORRECT ANSWERS)

1. CORRECT ANSWER: D (88)
   Convert 2.75 ft. to inches by multiplying by 12 = 33 in.
   Then, 33/.375 = 88

2. CORRECT ANSWER: E (None of the above)
   $1.50 is the price of a 6 oz. bar of chocolate.
   Since 1 lb. = 16 oz., the cost of 1 lb. of chocolate = $4.00 (16 × 2½).

3. CORRECT ANSWER: A (8)
   First, we must figure the number of feet that the man walks diagonally (AC in the diagram), and then we must find the number of feet that he will walk by going along the perimeter of the lot (from C to A by way of D, or CD + AD).
   Since the diagonal represented by x forms a right triangle, we have the equation:
   $x^2 = 50^2 + 120^2$ or $x^2 = 16,900$ x = 130 ft. (AC). CD + AD (walking along the perimeter) = 170 ft. (50+120).
   ∴ the man saves 4 ft. by walking diagonally (170-130); and since he walks at the rate of 5 ft. a second, he saves 8 sec. (40/5).

   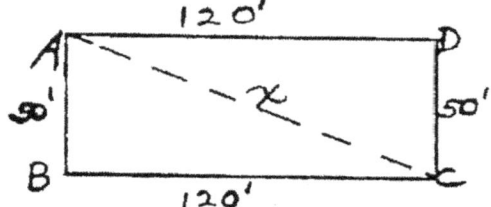

4. CORRECT ANSWER: B (40)
   Total time = 2 hours 52 min. or 172 min. (3:52 P.M. – 1 P.M.). Since there are 4 class periods, there are 3 intervals of 4 min. each (12 min. in all) between these periods.
   ∴ 172 – 12 = 160 min. (total time for the class periods) and 160/4 = 40 min. (time in each class period).

5. CORRECT ANSWER: C (3")
   Let x = length of the shorter dimension.
   ∴ $1^7/_8 : x = 2½ : 4$ or
   5/2x = 60/8 or 40x = 120, x = 3"

6. CORRECT ANSWER: B (2°)
   The sum of the temperatures given = 16; the number of readings is 7.
   ∴ 16°/7 = $2^2/_7$° or 2° (to the nearest degree)

7. CORRECT ANSWER: A (.94")
   Since the diameter of a circle is twice the radius, the outer radius is 7.19" (14.38"/2), and the inner radius is 6.25" (12.5÷2).
   ∴ the thickness of the pipe = .94" (7.19 – 6.25).

8. CORRECT ANSWER: B ($16^2/_3\%$)
   $4.40 + .50($4.40) = $6.60 (price as of February 2013).
   Since the ceiling price was announced as $5.50, a reduction of $1.10 was necessary ($6.60 - $5.50).
   ∴ $1.10 ÷ $6.60 = $\frac{1}{6}$ = $16^2/_3\%$.

9. CORRECT ANSWER: B (5)
   In computing square root, we group the digits by two's, beginning with the decimal point and moving by two's to the left. Since there are 5 groups of two, each of which will have 1 digit in the answer, there will be 5 digits.

10. CORRECT ANSWER: E (None of the above)
    Let x = time required for 6 tractors
    ∴ 4:6 (tractors) = x:12 (time) or
    6x = 48, x = 8 hours

EXAMINATION SECTION
TEST 1

DIRECTIONS: Each question or incomplete statement is followed by several suggested answers or completions. Select the one that *BEST* answers the question or completes the statement. *PRINT THE LETTER OF THE CORRECT ANSWER IN THE SPACE AT THE RIGHT.*

1. Of the following, the most important source of nitrogen compounds for green plants is   1._____

    A. nitrogen-rich rock particles
    B. lightning discharges
    C. nitrogen-fixing bacteria
    D. soil ammonia

2. The "all-or-none" reaction refers to which one of the following   2._____

    A. secretion of adrenalin
    B. transmission of the nerve impulse
    C. secretion of insulin
    D. digestion of carbohydrates

3. The center for temperature regulation in the human is the   3._____

    A. skin   B. lungs
    C. thalamus   D. medulla

4. Of the following, the most widespread motivation for behavior is the maintenance of   4._____

    A. the species   B. nutrition
    C. stability   D. instinctive patterns

5. The catastrophic "red tides" which kill many fish are most directly caused by   5._____

    A. depletion of the supply of oxygen
    B. increase in the mean temperature of the water
    C. the "bloom" of a certain dinoflagellate
    D. interference with metabolite equilibrium

6. Of the following, the term that is most closely associated with the microenvironment of a particular species is   6._____

    A. microclimate   B. niche
    C. community   D. biome

7. The swarming and breeding rhythm of palolo worms and grunions are affected mainly by the   7._____

    A. temperature of the water   B. availability of food
    C. lunar cycles and tides   D. density of the population

8. The pacemaker of the human heart is known as the   8._____

    A. bundle of His   B. mitral valve
    C. semilunar valve   D. sino-auricular node

9. A mutual partnership of two kinds of organisms is best exemplified by which one of the following?

   A. lichen
   B. legume
   C. liverwort
   D. limpet

10. Of the following, the nutrients that enter the human bloodstream at the thoracic duct are the

    A. amino acids
    B. fatty acids
    C. glucose
    D. vitamins

11. Analysis by chromatography has demonstrated

    A. the amino acids present in some proteins
    B. the taxonomic relationships among protists
    C. the ATP-content of some cell organelles
    D. mutagenic changes in the DNA molecule

12. Of the following, the organism that moves by means of a single flagellum is a/an

    A. colpidium
    B. euglena
    C. euplotes
    D. paramecium

13. Of the following hormones, the one that is most directly associated with the maintenance of pregnancy is

    A. insulin
    B. progestin
    C. secretin
    D. somatotrophin

14. A pupil treated guppies with a hormone and found that the normally dull-colored females developed bright colors. The hormone was most probably

    A. androgen
    B. estradiol
    C. pitocin
    D. thyroxin

15. Of the following, the organism that is now no longer classified as a rodent is the

    A. beaver
    B. capybara
    C. rabbit
    D. rat

16. Of the following, the substance that is LEAST closely related to amino acids is

    A. cortisone
    B. fibrinogen
    C. insulin
    D. thyroxin

17. Pollination characteristically occurs among which one of the following pairs?

    A. Angiosperms and psilopsids
    B. Angiosperms and gymnosperms
    C. Pteridophytes and bryophytes
    D. Bryophytes and angiosperms

18. Which one of the following is an early step in the photolytic reaction in plants?

    A. Splitting of carbon dioxide
    B. Splitting of chlorophyll

C. Ionization of carbon dioxide
D. Ionization of chlorophyll

19. Many plants store proteins in the form of which one of the following structures?

    A. Elaioplasts
    B. Starch grains
    C. Chromoplasts
    D. Aleurone grains

20. Of the following animals, the one in which true radial symmetry is found is

    A. starfish
    B. jellyfish
    C. shellfish
    D. silverfish

21. Of the following, the radioactive thorium-lead series would be most useful in determining the age of

    A. coprolites related to the Inca civilization
    B. an amphora
    C. tree fern fossils
    D. australopithecus

22. Recent evidence indicates that when myofibrils change in length, some of their constituent filamentous molecules

    A. slide past one another
    B. become coiled like a tight helix
    C. uncoil like a loose spiral
    D. fold like an accordion

23. The ending of metaphase may be marked by the splitting of the

    A. chromatids
    B. chromosomes
    C. kinetochores
    D. spindle fibres

24. Among the following, the first plants to reappear in a badly burned forest area will most probably be

    A. mosses
    B. ferns
    C. grasses
    D. dandelions

25. The "vagus substance" discovered by Loewi later turned out to be

    A. choline esterase
    B. adrenaline
    C. 5-hydroxytryptamine
    D. acetylcholine

26. According to normal genetic prediction a color blind girl ($X^c X^c$) must have had a father whose genetic makeup was

    A. $X^C X^c$
    B. $X^n Y^C$
    C. $X^c Y^c$
    D. $X^c Y$

27. Of the following, the vitamin most closely associated with carbohydrate metabolism is vitamin

    A. A
    B. B_1
    C. C
    D. D

28. Of the following, the type of enzyme most closely associated with cellular respiration is

    A. dehydrogenase
    B. lipase
    C. sucrase
    D. transaminase

29. If a dihybrid cross gives a phenotypic ratio of 9 : 3 : 3 : 1, this is proof of

    A. autosomal linkage
    B. heterosomal linkage
    C. non-linkage
    D. sex linkage

30. Of the following crosses, the one that is most likely to produce the largest number of recessive offspring is

    A. AA x Aa
    B. Aa x Aa
    C. Aa x aa
    D. AA x aa

31. An excretory structure that is typically found in planarians is the

    A. nephron
    B. flame cell
    C. Malpighian tubule
    D. nephridium

32. The ornithine cycle is a biochemical pathway which results in the production of

    A. ammonia
    B. ornithine
    C. urea
    D. ATP

33. Most substances pass through a plasma membrane by a process known as

    A. osmosis
    B. diffusion
    C. active transport
    D. passive transport

34. One way in which molecules that are too large to pass through a cell membrane can enter a cell is the process of

    A. transduction
    B. pinocytosis
    C. translocation
    D. transmigration

35. Clusters of proteins or protein-like substances that are held together within a surrounding liquid to form small droplets are called

    A. coacervates
    B. peptides
    C. conglomerates
    D. macroproteins

36. The destruction of coyotes because they may prey on sheep often results in the

    A. large-scale increase in the numbers of sheep
    B. starvation of sheep in competition with rabbits
    C. increase in the quality of mutton
    D. increase in diseases of sheep

37. The nature of a climax community is ultimately decided mainly by which one of the following?

    A. Initial flora
    B. Initial fauna
    C. Rate of succession
    D. Climate

38. A section of the circulatory system which plays an important role in fishes, but which disappears in higher land animals is the

   A. hepatic portal system
   B. renal portal system
   C. renal arteries
   D. hepatic arteries

39. The results of experimental grafting of tobacco shoots on tomato roots, and tomato shoots on tobacco roots gives evidence that

   A. only tobacco roots manufacture nicotine
   B. the leaves of the scion manufacture nicotine
   C. materials are transported upward only in the xylem
   D. some unrelated plants can be grafted together

40. Supplementary diverticula which help to increase the surface of the digestive tracts of fishes are called

   A. vermiform appendix
   B. colic caeca
   C. villi
   D. pyloric caeca

41. The one group of scientists, among the following, most closely associated with the Heterotroph Theory of the origin of life is

   A. Oparin, Miller, Urey
   B. Darwin, DeVries, Morgan
   C. Gamow, Wald, Crick
   D. Hyman, Romer, Szent-Gyorgyi

42. Companion-cells are most closely associated with which one of the following groups?

   A. Tracheids
   B. Vessels
   C. Gametes
   D. Sieve-tubes

43. When a Paramecium undergoes binary fission

   A. both micronucleus and macronucleus divide mitotically
   B. only the micronucleus divides mitotically
   C. only the macronucleus divides mitotically
   D. the micronucleus disintegrates

44. The discovery that the human chromosome number was 46 came as the result of using which one of the following pairs of cytological techniques?

   A. Chromatography and electron microscopy
   B. X-ray diffraction studies and ultraviolet microscopy
   C. Action of colchicine and treatment with hypotonic saline solution
   D. Fluorescein dyes and human tissue cultures

45. It is now believed that the first organ, among the following to produce antibody-producing cells in the development of the human body is the

   A. hypophysis
   B. spleen
   C. liver
   D. thymus

46. The skin color of the earliest men was probably

   A. white
   B. yellow
   C. black
   D. variable

47. Although diversity of organisms, as shown by the fossil record, generally increases with time, virtually every animal phylum was reduced in diversity during the period known as the

    A. Cambrian
    B. Silurian
    C. Carboniferous
    D. Triassic

48. The evolutionary development of the phyla of animals can best be represented as which one of the following?

    A. Ladder
    B. Web
    C. Fan
    D. Chain

49. The second law of thermodynamics is best illustrated by the

    A. flow of materials in a cycle
    B. flow of energy in a food chain
    C. maintenance of oxygen in the atmosphere
    D. maintenance of nitrogen compounds in the soil

50. Dwarfs seen in circuses are usually the result primarily of which one of the following?

    A. A defective thyroid gland
    B. Pituitary deficiency
    C. Inadequate diet
    D. Inheritance of genes for short limbs

KEY (CORRECT ANSWERS)

1. C	11. A	21. C	31. B	41. A
2. B	12. B	22. A	32. C	42. D
3. C	13. B	23. C	33. C	43. B
4. C	14. A	24. A	34. B	44. C
5. C	15. C	25. D	35. A	45. D
6. B	16. A	26. D	36. B	46. D
7. C	17. B	27. B	37. D	47. D
8. D	18. D	28. A	38. B	48. C
9. A	19. D	29. C	39. A	49. B
10. B	20. B	30. C	40. D	50. D

TEST 2

DIRECTIONS: Each question or incomplete statement is followed by several suggested answers or completions. Select the one that BEST answers the question or completes the statement. PRINT THE LETTER OF THE CORRECT ANSWER IN THE SPACE AT THE RIGHT.

1. The role of receptor organs in the body is to

    A. transmit impulses to the spinal cord
    B. transform stimuli into nerve impulses
    C. mediate nervous reactions
    D. act as reflex centers

    1.____

2. Of the following, which one of the pituitary hormones mainly controls the rate of androgen secretion?

    A. ACTH
    B. FSH
    C. GH
    D. LH

    2.____

3. Continuous, quantitative, genetic variations can best be accounted for by which one of the following?

    A. Independent assortment
    C. Multiple factors
    B. Environmental effects
    D. Blending inheritance

    3.____

4. The total number of genes contained by the four chromosomes of Drosophilia is estimated to be closest to which one of the following?

    A. 1,000
    C. 10,000
    B. 30,000
    D. 50,000

    4.____

5. Pleiotropy refers to the fact that

    A. many genes may affect a single character
    B. one gene may affect many characters
    C. series of genes may act as modifiers
    D. genes may act in an additive manner

    5.____

6. The concept that the DNA content of an egg holds the information needed to control its development agrees most closely with the

    A. vitalism
    C. preformation
    B. teleology
    D. epigenesis

    6.____

7. Of the following, the one which is an intermediate product formed before glucose in photosynthesis is

    A. ATP
    C. PGAL
    B. DPN
    D. TPN

    7.____

8. Solutions of crystal violet, iodine and alcohol are used in a staining procedure known as

    A. acid-fast stain
    C. Giemsa's stain
    B. Wright's stain
    D. Gram stain

    8.____

9. One stage of the life history of Plasmodium is spent as which one of the following?

    A. Oocyst in the body of a human
    B. Trophozoite in the body of Anopheles
    C. Merozoite in the body of man
    D. Gametocyte in the salivary gland of Anopheles

10. The first sound of the heart beat is produced when

    A. the auriculo-ventricular valves snap shut to prevent backflow of blood into the auricles
    B. the valves in the aorta and pulmonary arteries snap shut to prevent backflow into the ventricles
    C. the auricles fill suddenly with returning blood
    D. the blood spurts forward in the aorta and pulmonary arteries

11. Position in crayfish is determined by sand grains resting on sensitive cells in the ampullae. If these grains are replaced by iron particles and a magnet is held over the the crayfish, the animal will

    A. remain right side up   B. turn to the right
    C. turn to the left   D. turn upside down

12. After hatching, an 8 hour old chick will follow the first moving object it sees and behave as if the object were its mother. This phenomenon is known as

    A. reflex behavior   B. conditioning
    C. imprinting   D. instinctive behavior

13. Of the following, the stage that is MOST closely associated with the replication of chromosomes and DNA is

    A. reduction division stage of meiosis
    B. anaphase of mitosis
    C. interphase and prophase of mitosis
    D. fertilization

14. At which one of the following sites are amino acids assembled to form proteins?

    A. Pinocytes   B. Nucleolar RNA
    C. Plasmagenes   D. Ribosomal RNA

15. Ferns, conifers, and flowering plants are classified as

    A. Tracheophyta   B. Spermatophyta
    C. Psilophyta   D. Chlorophyta

16. Most of the oxidative enzymes of the cell and of the tricarboxylic acid cycle are concentrated within which one of the following?

    A. Grana of chloroplasts   B. Cristae of mitochondria
    C. Ergastoplasm   D. Golgi apparatus

17. In the life history of a moss, reduction division occurs in the

    A. sporophyte generation   B. gametophyte generation
    C. antheridia and archegonia   D. seeds

18. The fruit composed of a hard endocarp and usually one seed is classified as which one of the following?

   A. Capsule
   B. Drupe
   C. Achene
   D. Samara

19. Active ciliary action can most easily be demonstrated under the microscope by using a wet mount of which one of the following?

   A. Conjugating paramecium
   B. Epidermis of frog's mouth
   C. Epithelium of rat jejanum
   D. Live euglena

20. Of the following the most convenient way to prepare to show a class live zygospores is to order

   A. a freshly collected mass of Spirogyra
   B. cultured Oedogonium
   C. fresh yeast and a dilute molasses solution
   D. plus and minus strain spores of Rhizopus nigricans

21. The sweet pea blossom is a good example of a self-pollinating plant because of the structure called the

   A. keel
   B. epigynous ovary
   C. bract
   D. spathe

22. Of the following, a normal function of the human kidney is that it

   A. allows excess amino acids in the glomerulus to filter into the urine
   B. reabsorbs nitrogenous compounds when their concentration in the blood plasma falls below a critical level
   C. reabsorbs less water than it eliminates
   D. reabsorbs more water than it eliminates

23. Of the following hormones the one that does NOT strongly influence the level of blood sugar is

   A. glucagon
   B. intermedin
   C. ACTH
   D. thyroxin

24. Some of the largest and oldest trees of the earth occur, in the United States, in the biogeographic zone known as the

   A. southeastern evergreen forests
   B. eastern coniferous forest
   C. Rocky Mountain coniferous forest
   D. Pacific coastal coniferous forest

25. A blood vessel that is functional during development of mammals but normally becomes closed at birth is the

   A. duct of Cuvier
   B. ductus arteriosis
   C. foramen ovale
   D. thoracic duct

26. Which one of the following is a technique that is used to separate mitochondria from other cellular fractions?

   A. Mass spectrography
   B. Differential centrifugation
   C. Gas chromatography
   D. Partition chromatography

27. According to currently accepted theory, in the evolution of life, primary heterotrophs were probably preceded by which one of the following?

   A. Photosynthetic autotrophs
   B. A period of organic synthesis
   C. Virus-like organisms
   D. Primitive aerobic aggregates

28. The human defect called "Mongolian mental deficiency" is caused by

   A. accumulation of phenylpyruvic acid
   B. anoxia during pregnancy
   C. trisomic condition of one autosome
   D. defective DNA in X chromosomes

29. In both taxonomic and evolutionary studies, homologous structures are significant because they may indicate

   A. structural diversity   B. functional similarity
   C. genetic relationship   D. genetic diversity

30. Of the following organisms, the one that has an incomplete, but functional, digestive system is

   A. Lumbricus   B. Lobster
   C. Planaria   D. Grasshopper

31. In the rabbit and rat, as contrasted with man, the smallest area of the cerebral cortex is concerned with

   A. sensory function   B. motor function
   C. somatic sensation   D. association

32. A microscopic slide preparation of unstained young elodea leaf is an excellent source for demonstrating

   A. cilia in plants   B. cyclosis
   C. mitosis   D. stomata

33. During replication the strands of the DNA molecule separate to form 2 complementary strands at the bond linkage of

   A. oxygen   B. hydrogen
   C. nitrogen   D. carbon

34. The synapses of the pre and post ganglionic fibers of the parasympathetic system are located at which one of the following sites?

    A. Just outside the spinal cord
    B. In the chain ganglia
    C. Close to the internal organs
    D. In the solar plexus

35. Hybrid vigor probably is a result of

    A. eliminating the homozygous condition of most pairs of genes
    B. decreasing the number of heterozygous pairs
    C. stimulating the process of heteropycnosis
    D. increasing the number of beneficial mutations

36. Of the following, the vitamin that forms part of two co-enzyme systems, DPN and TNP, is

    A. ascorbic acid   B. biotin
    C. riboflavin   D. nicotinamide

37. In a cross between two roan short horn cattle, the progeny resulting should show white, colored, and roan in the ratio of

    A. 1 : 2 : 1   B. 12 : 3 : 1
    C. 9 : 3 : 3 : 1   D. 1 : 1 : 1

38. Of the following sources, the most convincing evidence that DNA is the genetic material comes from studies on

    A. bacteria and viruses   B. protozoa
    C. Drosophila   D. molds

39. Progesterone is secreted by the

    A. pituitary   B. wall of the uterus
    C. corpus lutum   D. placenta

40. Much of the phenomena of tropistic responses of plants to light were first observed by which one of the following?

    A. Charles Darwin   B. Jacques Loeb
    C. Ivan Pavlov   D. Lloyd Morgan

41. Dying, abnormally distorted bacterial cells are often referred to as

    A. ghost forms   B. involution forms
    C. retrograde forms   D. bacteriolytic forms

42. Tularemia is a disease caused by a(n)

    A. gramnegative bacillus B. wild rodent
    C. small virus   D. amoeba-like protozoan

43. Of the following, the pairs which are examples of complex organic compounds with high energy bonds are

    A. DNA, ATP   B. DDT, 2,4-D
    C. RNA, DNA   D. ATP, ADP

44. Of the following, the condition under which a stomatal pore will open is when the

    A. turgor of the guard cells decreases
    B. turgor of the guard cells increases
    C. leaf is kept in the dark
    D. amount of CO_2 in the guard cells increases

45. Using a conventional microscope, one can gauge the thickness of a cell by manipulating

    A. the iris periphery
    B. the condenser and oil immersion objective
    C. the stage micrometer
    D. the fine adjustment wheel

46. Of the following, which one is the control center for the knee jerk reflex?

    A. Semicircular canals   B. Hypothalamus
    C. Medulla   D. Spinal cord

47. Which one of the following would best explain why prolonged use of antibiotics may result in a deficiency of vitamin K?

    A. Dietary vitamin K is restored
    B. Absorption of vitamin K is blocked
    C. The bacterial flora of the intestine is changed
    D. Digestion of fats is impeded

48. Many of the enzymes that function during cellular respiration are closely associated with which one of the following parts of a cell?

    A. Golgi apparatus   B. Mitochondria
    C. Trichocysts   D. pinocytic vesicles

49. Fossil evidence has decisively shown that the origin of the camel was in which one of the following regions?

    A. Outer Mongolia   B. Syria
    C. Australia   D. North America

50. Of the following, the basic function of the contractile vacuole in a paramecium is

    A. hydrophilic   B. sclerotic
    C. hydrostatic   D. electrophoretic

KEY (CORRECT ANSWERS)

1. B	11. D	21. A	31. D	41. B
2. D	12. C	22. D	32. B	42. A
3. C	13. C	23. B	33. B	43. D
4. B	14. D	24. D	34. C	44. B
5. B	15. A	25. B	35. A	45. D
6. D	16. B	26. B	36. D	46. D
7. C	17. A	27. B	37. A	47. C
8. D	18. B	28. C	38. A	48. B
9. C	19. B	29. C	39. C	49. D
10. A	20. D	30. C	40. A	50. C

TEST 3

DIRECTIONS: Each question or incomplete statement is followed by several suggested answers or completions. Select the one that BEST answers the question or completes the statement. PRINT THE LETTER OF THE CORRECT ANSWER IN THE SPACE AT THE RIGHT.

1. The Hardy-Weinberg law refers to phenomena related to

   A. population genetics
   B. intermediary hydrotropism
   C. bacterial conduction
   D. cytological biochemistry

2. Of the following blood vessels, the ones MOST responsible for determining how much blood flows through organs are the

   A. small arteries B. arterioles
   C. capillaries   D. venules

3. Bilateral embryonic symmetry and an apparent radial adult symmetry is illustrated in the phylum of which one of the following?

   A. Mollusks   B. Coelenterates
   C. Chordates   D. Echinoderms

4. Of the following, the photosensitive visual pigment that functions best when there is a plentiful supply of dietary vitamin A is

   A. chlorophyll B. porphyrin
   C. chromatin   D. rhodopsin

5. The principle that best explains the rise of fluids in a Sequoia tree is that of

   A. the sodium pump   B. positive atmospheric pressure
   C. transpiration and cohesion   D. meiosis

6. The abscission of leaves adapts trees to

   A. manufacture gibberellins
   B. conserve water
   C. repel rodents
   D. grow faster during the cold season

7. Most lumber that is ordinarily used commercially is derived from

   A. heartwood B. dogwood
   C. lenticels D. cork cambium

8. The conveyance of which one of the following is a function of human blood but NOT a function of grasshopper blood?

   A. Nutrients B. Oxygen
   C. Hormones   D. Wastes

9. The loop of Henle is associated with the

   A. brain B. kidney
   C. pancreas D. large intestine

10. The concentration of urea is greatest in the

    A. hepatic artery B. hepatic portal vein
    C. hepatic vein D. hepatic duct

11. Which one of the following is NOT a hormone?

    A. auxin B. ACTH
    C. indoleacetic acid D. riboflavin

12. The trait among the following that appears to be sex-linked in humans is

    A. eye color B. Rh factor
    C. ability to taste mannose D. hemophilia

13. Beriberi is a deficiency disease caused by a lack of

    A. minerals B. nitrates
    C. thiamin D. carbohydrates

14. Which one of the following pairs is composed of the two unrelated members?

    A. Sea cucumber—sea lily B. Horseshoe crab—octopus
    C. Nautilus—garden slug D. Scallop—squid

15. Cholecystokinin is a hormone that

    A. is produced in the bile
    B. stimulates contraction of the urinary bladder
    C. antagonizes secretin
    D. is produced in the duodenum

16. Which one of the following is a gas whose concentration in inspired air is about the same as it is in expired air?

    A. Hydrogen B. Carbon dioxide
    C. Nitrogen D. Oxygen

17. Loewi's experiment with frog hearts led to the discovery of

    A. adrenalin B. nor-epinephrin
    C. acetylcholine D. pentaquine

18. The beginning of tetany is due to an undersecretion by which one of these glands?

    A. Thyroid B. Parathyroid
    C. Ductless D. Pancreas

19. Of the following, the one which is a living organism from which it is possible to obtain flagellates capable of digesting cellulose is the

    A. crow B. rabbit C. mite D. squirrel

20. In which one of the following plant regions do gibberellins most stimulate growth?

   A. Heartwood
   B. Roots
   C. Buds
   D. Stem internodes

21. Of the following, the one who was a pioneer in the investigation of plant hormones was

   A. Went
   B. Funk
   C. Rowntree
   D. Gabrielson

22. An eosinophil is identified as a

   A. type of cell in the gastric mucosa
   B. red blood corpuscle
   C. white blood corpuscle
   D. type of neurone

23. Which one of the following descriptions does NOT fit an amoeba?

   A. Regions of solation and gelation are visible
   B. Amitotic division is the normal method of reproduction
   C. Pseudopods are extended during locomotion
   D. It has a nucleus that can be excised with proper instruments

24. If a biologist wishes to observe the chromosome changes in a living cell dividing by mitosis, which one of the following microscopes should he use?

   A. Compound light
   B. Stereoscopic binocular
   C. Phase-contrast
   D. Electrostatic

25. Of the following, the one which is an organism that is especially suitable for demonstrating giant chromosomes is the

   A. trochophore larva
   B. bipinnaria larva
   C. drosophila larva
   D. hydrophyte larva

26. Stimulation of the vagus nerve will cause

   A. secretion of gastric juice
   B. dilation of the eustachian tubes
   C. inhibition of metabolism
   D. an increase in the heart beat

27. Assuming that the limit of resolving power of the human eye is one tenth of a millimeter, which one of the following cells would just be visible to the unaided human eye under ordinary conditions of light?

   A. White blood cell (5 microns)
   B. Paramecium (250 microns)
   C. Human egg cell (100 microns)
   D. Amoeba (600 microns)

28. A series of hydrogen acceptors is found mainly in which one of the following?

   A. Water vacuoles of protozoa
   B. Capsule of Bowman

C. Digestive system
D. Cytochrome system of cellular enzymes

29. When a maltose molecule is digested into two molecules of glucose, the process is called hydrolysis because

   A. water is added to the maltose molecule
   B. water is removed from the maltose molecule
   C. water dissolves the glucose molecules
   D. water and glucose are products

30. Of the following, the one which is an example of a buffer system in blood is

   A. hemoglobin and oxyhemoglobin
   B. oxygen and carbon dioxide
   C. albumin and globulin
   D. sodium bicarbonate and carbonic acid

31. The heart muscle receives its nutrition and oxygen from the blood in the

   A. ventricles   B. auricles
   C. septum   D. coronary artery

32. When bronchioles are obstructed, fresh oxygen is most directly kept from reaching the

   A. bronchial tubes   B. alveolar capillaries
   C. larynx   D. trachea

33. Syncytial units are found in which one of the following human tissues?

   A. Striated muscle   B. Nerve
   C. Cartilage   D. Epithelial

34. As a result of experiments with radioactive isotopes, it has been determined that replication of chromosomes occurs during

   A. prophase   B. metaphase
   C. interphase D. anaphase

35. Of the following, the cellular structure noted for protein synthesis is the

   A. pinocytic vesicle   B. ribosome
   C. lysosome   D. chondriosome

36. The observation that alcohol and ether readily penetrate the membrane of cells suggests that the plasma membrane consists partly of layers of

   A. glucose   B. lipid
   C. starch   D. amino-acids

37. Of the following characteristics, the one relevant to trace elements is that they

   A. are radioactive and can be located with a Geiger Counter
   B. exist in minute amounts in protoplasm
   C. are not readily absorbed into protoplasm
   D. act as inhibitors of enzymatic reactions

38. Of the following statements concerning transfer of organic compounds and ions across membranes, the one which is NOT correct is that it

    A. occurs against a concentration gradient
    B. follows a concentration gradient
    C. requires energy
    D. is inhibited by dinitrophenol that hydrolyzes ATP

39. The pH optimum of gastric juice is about

    A. 1.5-2   B. 3.5-4
    C. 5.5-6   D. 7.5-8

40. When red corpuscles are placed in a hypotonic salt solution, they

    A. undergo hemolysis
    B. form rouleaux
    C. undergo normoblastic activity
    D. become crenated

41. Which one of the following BEST describes a nerve impulse?

    A. The cessation of an electric current
    B. A chemical flow throughout the nerve fiber
    C. Synaptic secretion of acetylcholine
    D. A wave of electrical depolarization

42. Of the following organisms, the one that may live as an autotroph or heterotroph is

    A. Euglena   B. Blepharisma
    C. Fucus   D. Paramecium

43. All of the following are characteristic of a tundra EXCEPT that

    A. it is a vast northern zone encircling the Artic Ocean
    B. it is an extensive zone in the Southern Hemisphere
    C. there are no upstanding trees on it, but only dwarf conifers, willows and birches
    D. ptarmigans, flies, snow shoe hare, and caribou are numerous on it

44. Which one of the following gives the varieties of trees present normally in a climax forest common to much of the northeastern United States?

    A. Ponderosa pine   B. Beech and maple forest
    C. Pine and oak   D. Oak and tulip trees

45. Pyrenoids are associated with which one of the following?

    A. mitochondria   B. nuclei
    C. chloroplasts   D. ribosomes

46. Phylum Tracheophyta includes which one of the following sets?

    A. Mosses and ferns
    B. Ferns and flowering plants
    C. True fungi and flowering plants
    D. Liverworts, club mosses, and mosses

47. To which one of the following choices can many plant movements best be attributed?

   A. Auxins
   B. Kinetins
   C. Contractile substances
   D. A combination of turgor and growth differentials

48. Which one of the following wavelengths of light, if withheld from a geranium plant would limit the rate of photosynthesis?

   A. Red   B. Green   C. Orange   D. Ultraviolet

49. For which one of the following processes is an appropriate photo-period necessary?

   A. The onset of pollination
   B. The onset of flowering
   C. The onset of vernalization
   D. Osmosis

50. Adding ribonuclease to cells would effectively inhibit which one of the following processes?

   A. Protein synthesis
   B. Diffusion
   C. Catalysis
   D. Lipogenesis

KEY (CORRECT ANSWERS)

1. A	11. D	21. A	31. D	41. D
2. B	12. D	22. C	32. B	42. A
3. D	13. C	23. B	33. A	43. B
4. D	14. B	24. C	34. C	44. B
5. C	15. D	25. C	35. B	45. C
6. B	16. C	26. A	36. B	46. B
7. A	17. C	27. C	37. B	47. A
8. B	18. B	28. D	38. B	48. A
9. B	19. A	29. A	39. A	49. B
10. C	20. D	30. D	40. A	50. A

TEST 4

DIRECTIONS: Each question or incomplete statement is followed by several suggested answers or completions. Select the one that BEST answers the question or completes the statement. PRINT THE LETTER OF THE CORRECT ANSWER IN THE SPACE AT THE RIGHT.

1. A blue methylene blue solution placed in a tissue culture medium will become bleached if the tissue is undergoing which one of the following?

    A. Hydrolysis
    B. Deaminization
    C. Hydrogenation
    D. Dehydrogenation

2. Of the following, the one that is a cellular enzyme that is involved in the production of pigment is

    A. acetyl coenzyme A
    B. acetyl cholinesterase
    C. tyrosinase
    D. ribonuclease

3. A drop of type B blood will clump in

    A. both anti-A and anti-B serum
    B. neither anti-A nor anti-B serum
    C. anti-A serum but not anti-B serum
    D. anti-B serum but not anti-A serum

4. The concept of the "constancy of the internal environment" is attributed to

    A. Claude Bernard
    B. Louis Pasteur
    C. Arthur Sherrington
    D. Linus Pauling

5. Vitamin K is the precursor of

    A. thrombin
    B. thrombokinase
    C. thromboplastin
    D. prothrombin

6. Which one of the following is an intermediate product of metabolism that cells can convert to protein, fat, or carbohydrate?

    A. Vitamin K
    B. Pyruvic acid
    C. Carbonic acid
    D. Glucose-6-phosphate

7. Hemoglobin is to Fe as chlorophyll is to

    A. Zn
    B. Mg
    C. Mn
    D. Al

8. Of the following, the phylum of worms that is of economic importance because of the damage done by its members to crops is

    A. the annelids
    B. the platyhelminthes
    C. the nematodes
    D. the acanthocephalans

9. Anerobic oxidation in both yeast cells and muscle cells is equivalent to

    A. the Krebs cycle
    B. photosynthetic phosphorylation

186

C. oxidation by the cytochrome system
D. fermentation

10. Of the following, the compound that is closely associated with the contraction of muscle fibers is   10._____

   A. actinomycin   B. actomyosin
   C. nigrosin   D. interferon

11. Recent research has shown that the thymus gland plays an important role in   11._____

   A. antigen-antibody reactions
   B. antigen-antibiotic reactions
   C. hormone release
   D. digestive reactions

12. Genes are to chromosomes as grana are to   12._____

   A. mitochondria   B. chloroplasts
   C. Golgi bodies   D. amyloplasts

13. The timing of bird migration appears to be controlled by   13._____

   A. geocentric lines of force
   B. temperature
   C. availability of food
   D. endocrine glands that respond to changes in the length of the day

14. The experiments of Dr. Lorenz provided evidence that the attraction of newly hatched ducklings to the mother is which one of the following?   14._____

   A. Inherited   B. Instinctive
   C. Imprinted   D. Tropistic

15. Which one of the following compounds stores energy that is immediately available for active muscle cells?   15._____

   A. Creatine phosphate   B. Glycogen
   C. Glucose   D. Glycine

16. The hormone which has an effect similar to that of the stimulation of the entire sympathetic nervous system is   16._____

   A. pituitrin   B. thyroxin
   C. insulin   D. adrenalin

17. The regulation of body temperature in man is controlled by the   17._____

   A. medulla   B. cerebellum
   C. hypothalamus   D. pons

18. Which one of the following BEST illustrates instinctive behavior?   18._____

   A. Blinking of the eyes
   B. The solving of a maze by a rat
   C. Jumping at a sudden noise
   D. The spinning of a spider web

19. Which one of the following would a rat NOT be able to do if its cerebellum were destroyed

   A. Digest food
   B. Breathe
   C. Walk
   D. Hear

20. Sexuality has been demonstrated in all of the following EXCEPT

   A. Chlorella
   B. yeasts
   C. Paramecium
   D. bacteria

21. The anti-Rh antibody is produced in the mother's blood in which one of the following cases?

   A. Rh negative woman bearing an Rh positive child
   B. Rh negative woman bearing an Rh negative child
   C. Rh positive woman bearing an Rh negative child
   D. Hybrid Rh positive woman bearing an Rh negative child

22. The part of the brain that has a function similar to that of the semicircular canals is the

   A. medulla
   B. cerebellum
   C. cerebrum
   D. hypothalamus

23. When large numbers of "blue" Andalusian fowl are crossed, which one of the following represents a possible distribution of progeny?

   A. 100% blue
   B. 75% blue, 25% white
   C. 25% black, 50% blue, 25% white
   D. 50% black, 50% white

24. To determine whether a "black" guinea pig is pure black or hybrid black, it should be crossed with which one of the following kinds of guinea pigs?

   A. White
   B. Pure black
   C. Hybrid white
   D. An unknown

25. One stock of fruit flies having black bodies and vestigial wings can be used to show which one of the following?

   A. Linkage
   B. Sex linkage
   C. Complementary genes
   D. Supplementary genes

26. The most frequent of the following blood groups in humans is

   A. A
   B. B
   C. AB
   D. O

27. When two organisms, each hybrid for a given trait, are crossed, a large progeny will show which one of the following percentage of hybrids?

   A. 100%
   B. 75%
   C. 50%
   D. 25%

28. If a piece of a stalk of Acetabularia mediterranea is grafted onto the nucleus-containing rhizoid of Acetabularia crenulata, the cap produced will show the characteristics of

   A. Acetabularia mediterranea
   B. Acetabularia crenulata

C. both species of Acetabularia
D. neither species of Acetabularia

29. Of the following, the one which is an example of an inactive form of an enzyme is

    A. pepsinogen   B. coenzyme A
    C. gastrin   D. secretin

30. Sodium citrate is added to bottles of donor blood to prevent clotting because it removes the

    A. serum   B. fibrinogen
    C. calcium   D. prothrombin

31. Cellulose is digested in the rumen of cattle by the enzyme cellulase secreted by

    A. protozoa   B. bacteria
    C. the rumen   D. the esophagus

32. The main process that occurs in the dark reaction in photosynthesis is

    A. that water is split   B. that carbon dioxide is fixed
    C. that glucose is oxidized   D. the Hill reaction

33. Of the following possibilities, the evidence that untrained planaria worms, when fed chopped planarian worms which had learned a maze, were able to learn a maze faster than the controls, indicates that learning is

    A. associated with reflexes   B. associated with RNA
    C. an instinct   D. a conditioned activity

34. Of the following, the crop that would be MOST likely to deplete the soil of its nitrates is

    A. alfalfa   B. soybeans   C. clover   D. corn

35. To improve the quality of beef a breeder would probably use which one of the following methods?

    A. Selection   B. Inbreeding
    C. Hybridization   D. Parthenogenesis

36. A "Killer" trait in paramecium is associated with which one of the following?

    A. Nucleus and kappa   B. Nucleus and kinetin
    C. Cytoplasm   D. Trichocysts

37. Of the following, which one probably gives the correct succession of early man?

    A. Neanderthal ---- Piltdown ---- Sinanthropus
    B. Sinanthropus ---- Pithecanthropus
    C. Cro-Magnon ---- Neanderthal
    D. Pithecanthropus ---- Neanderthal ---- Cro-Magnon

38. The history of early man dates back to which one of these periods?

    A. Jurassic   B. Pleistocene
    C. Paleocene   D. Permian

39. The Feulgen reaction is specific for which one of the following?

    A. Cilia
    B. DNA
    C. Mitochondria
    D. Cytoplasm

40. Motile sperm cells are found in all of the following plants EXCEPT

    A. Pine
    B. Gingko
    C. Mosses
    D. Ferns

41. The "one gene-one enzyme" explanation of gene action was developed by

    A. Morgan & Muller
    B. Watson & Crick
    C. Sturtevant & Bridges
    D. Beadle & Tatum

42. Given that the ability to taste thiocarbamide (P.T.C.) is an inherited trait, if one parent is a hybrid "taster," and the six offspring show some "tasters" and some "non-tasters," then the other parent is probably

    A. a pure "taster"
    B. dihybrid
    C. hybrid "non-taster"
    D. a pure "non-taster"

43. If a heterozygous black, smooth-haired guinea pig is crossed to a white, heterozygous rough-haired mate, all of the following distributions would be in accordance with the laws of probability for a large number of progeny EXCEPT that

    A. 50% may have black hair
    B. 50% may have white hair; half of these may be smooth-haired, half may be rough-haired
    C. 75% may have black hair
    D. 50% may have rough-hair

44. Chromatids and chiasmata refer to stages in which one of the following?

    A. Cleavage
    B. Optic stimulation
    C. Meiosis
    D. Induction

45. A luciferin - luciferase system refers to which one of the following?

    A. Visual pigments in fish
    B. Photosynthesizing pigments of bacteria
    C. Transformation in bacteria
    D. Bioluminescence

46. In the frog the long yellow structure applied along the length of each kidney is the

    A. adrenal
    B. spleen
    C. vagus nerve
    D. testis

47. Plasma cells are specialized cells that produce which one of the following?

    A. Thrombocytes
    B. Antibodies
    C. Granulocytes
    D. Leucocytes

48. Of the following, the one which is an enzyme, in cells, that catalyzes the reaction
    $2 H_2O_2 \rightarrow 2 H_2O + O_2$ is

    A. lipase
    B. catalase
    C. phosphorylase
    D. invertase

49. The normal body temperature for man, in degrees Centigrade, is closest to which one of the following?

   A. 20   B. 27   C. 37   D. 98.6

50. It is probable that a mammal smaller than a shrew could NOT exist because it would
   A. not get sufficient oxygen
   B. reproduce too rapidly
   C. have to eat at too tremendous a rate
   D. not be able to defend itself

KEY (CORRECT ANSWERS)

1. D	11. A	21. A	31. B	41. D
2. C	12. B	22. B	32. B	42. D
3. D	13. D	23. C	33. B	43. C
4. A	14. C	24. A	34. D	44. C
5. D	15. A	25. A	35. C	45. D
6. B	16. D	26. D	36. A	46. A
7. B	17. C	27. C	37. D	47. B
8. C	18. D	28. B	38. B	48. B
9. D	19. C	29. A	39. B	49. C
10. B	20. A	30. C	40. A	50. C

TEST 5

DIRECTIONS: Each question or incomplete statement is followed by several suggested answers or completions. Select the one that *BEST* answers the question or completes the statement. *PRINT THE LETTER OF THE CORRECT ANSWER IN THE SPACE AT THE RIGHT.*

1. The tusks of the Proboscidea are modified

   A. premolars
   B. canines
   C. frontal skull bones
   D. incisors

   1.___

2. In general biogeographical evidence of evolution has shown that

   A. centers of dispersion of animals usually have the most advanced forms predominating
   B. the farther one gets from the center of dispersion the more variation is found in the species and genera
   C. geographic barriers usually result in the extinction of genera
   D. fossils rarely form in river valleys

   2.___

3. Archeopteryx is a link between the members of which one of the following pairs?

   A. Amphibian-bird
   B. Fish-amphibian
   C. Reptile-mammal
   D. Reptile-bird

   3.___

4. Of the following, the organism capable of everting a digestive organ is the

   A. sponge   B. squid   C. rotifer   D. starfish

   4.___

5. Serological tests of phylogenetic relationships have strengthened the view that the vertebrates are MOST closely associated with which one of the following?

   A. Peripatus
   B. King crabs
   C. Echinoderms
   D. Molluscs

   5.___

6. Fossils are *MOST* likely to be discovered in which one of the following?

   A. River valley deposits
   B. Granite
   C. Basalt
   D. Volcanic deposits

   6.___

7. Organisms that normally convert protein decomposition ammonia to other compounds generally

   A. have a terrestrial habitat or mode of life
   B. are plants
   C. are autochthonous
   D. occupy an aquatic habitat

   7.___

8. An organism lacking chlorophyll, but nevertheless able to carry out photosynthesis has been found among which one of the following?

   A. Bacteria
   B. Viruses
   C. Phaeophytes
   D. Zoophytes

   8.___

192

9. The category of protista includes the

   A. algae, fungi, and protozoa
   B. algae, fungi, and bryophytes
   C. fungi, bryophytes, and protozoa
   D. protozoa, bryophytes, and tracheophytes

10. A characteristic of all chordates is the presence of a

    A. chorda tympanum
    B. chorda tendonae
    C. notochord
    D. vertebral column

11. Free-floating microscopic marine algae are known as

    A. benthon
    B. chlorophytes
    C. nekton
    D. plankton

12. An insect that can transmit a disease producing organism from one host to another is called which one of the following?

    A. Commensal
    B. Symbiont
    C. Vector
    D. Saprophyte

13. Of the following diseases, the one that is caused by a parasitic worm is

    A. ringworm
    B. tetanus
    C. trichinosis
    D. typhus

14. The equation:

    $$6 CO_2 + 6 H_2O + \text{kinetic energy} \rightarrow C_6 H_{12} O_6 + 6 O_2$$

    represents which one of the following processes?

    A. Respiration
    B. Glycolysis
    C. Krebs cycle
    D. photosynthesis

15. When a patch of white hair is shaved from a Himalayan rabbit, the hair grows back black in color if the rabbit is maintained at a low temperature during this period of new growth of hair. This is due to the fact that the

    A. expression of a gene is a result of heredity and environment
    B. gene for white is recessive
    C. genes have mutated
    D. white is the phenotype, not the genotype

16. The gene for yellow in mice shows abnormal ratios in the offspring: Yellow x non-yellow produce yellow and non-yellow progeny in a 1 : 1 ratio; yellow x yellow produce yellows and non-yellows in a ratio of 2 : 1. This variation has been shown to be due to the fact that yellow is

    A. due to two pairs of genes
    B. lethal when homozygous
    C. a case of incomplete dominance
    D. due to a double recessive

17. Of the following, which one BEST describes phenylketonuria?

    A. A vitamin deficiency resulting in abnormal metabolism of proteins
    B. An inherited metabolic disorder resulting in a lack of an enzyme
    C. A mineral deficiency resulting in abnormal bone formation
    D. An abnormal shape in red blood cells

Notice that questions 18-20 are related.

18. When a large number of homozygous polled red bulls were mated to horned white cows, their offspring were polled roan. This would seem to indicate that

    A. polled is dominant and roan shows incomplete dominance
    B. polled and roan are linked traits
    C. polled is hybrid and roan is a pure trait
    D. the number of progeny is too small to determine whether roan shows incomplete dominance

19. Producing an F_2 from the progeny in the above question would result in which one of the following ratios?

    A. 9 : 3 : 3 : 1
    B. 1 : 2 : 1 : 3
    C. 3 : 6 : 3 : 1 : 2 : 1
    D. 13 : 1 : 2 : 1

20. The F_2 offspring of the cross of polled roan cattle referred to above give evidence of which one of the following?

    A. Epistasis
    B. Linkage
    C. Dominance
    D. Independent assortment

21. All of the following statements are at least partially descriptive of a freemartin EXCEPT that it is a

    A. heifer twin-born with a bull calf
    B. heifer that is sterile and shows a tendency toward maleness
    C. bull with extra set of Y chromosomes
    D. case showing that sex hormones affect development of early embryos

22. Of the following diseases, with which one was Semmelweis closely associated?

    A. Cholera
    B. Puerperal fever
    C. Yellow fever
    D. Anthrax

23. The technique for isolating bacteria by means of a solid medium was developed by which one of the following?

    A. Pasteur
    B. Koch
    C. Ehrlich
    D. Fleming

24. Which one of the following would NOT likely be captured from a pond by means of a net?

    A. Larvae of dragon flies
    B. Flatworms
    C. Fucus
    D. Elodea

25. Soil water moves upward in stems through the

   A. pith   B. phloem   C. xylem   D. cambium

26. The oxygen given off during photosynthesis is derived from

   A. carbon dioxide
   B. water
   C. both water and carbon dioxide
   D. neither water nor carbon dioxide

27. Of the following, the hormone in plants that is involved in tropisms is

   A. anthocyanin   B. auxin
   C. carotene   D. xanthophyll

28. Which one of the following plants is important in enriching the soil in the process of crop rotation?

   A. Corn   B. Clover   C. Squash   D. Tomatoes

29. The carbohydrate usually found in the cell walls of plant cells is

   A. cellulose   B. keratin
   C. linin   D. mucin

30. Which one of the following men is MOST closely associated with the study of genetics?

   A. Brown   B. Morgan
   C. Purkinje D. Wilson

31. Ladders have been constructed around dams for conservation of which one of the following?

   A. Beaver   B. Frogs   C. Otters   D. Salmon

32. Of the following, the one which is an example of a useful American animal that has become extinct because of bad conservation practices is the

   A. bison   B. dodo
   C. passenger pigeon D. southeastern opossum

33. Bile salts are necessary to permit the action of the enzyme known as

   A. secretin   B. steapsin
   C. trypsin   D. erepsin

34. Which one of the following vitamins has commonly been added to bread which is called "enriched"?

   A. Menadione   B. Calciferol   C. Thiamin   D. Carotene

35. Of the following, a characteristic of bone tissue is the presence of large numbers of

   A. canals   B. striations
   C. myofibrils   D. spindle fibers

36. The structure in a mammal in which the embryo develops is the

   A. uterus
   B. ureter
   C. urethra
   D. utriculus

37. Which one of the following reactions is inborn in man?

   A. Conditioned reflex
   B. Habit
   C. Simple reflex
   D. Tropism

38. Ploughing furrows around a hill, rather than up and down it, is called plowing on the

   A. contour   B. grade   C. level   D. syncline

39. Incompletely decayed organic matter on the undisturbed floor of a forest is called

   A. loam
   B. topsoil
   C. humus
   D. peat moss

40. Which one of the following BEST typifies the expression, "universal currency of energy exchange"?

   A. DNA   B. FSH   C. PTC   D. ATP

41. Which one of the following contains guanine, cytosine, adenine, and thymine?

   A. ACTH   B. ATP   C. DNA   D. ADP

42. Which one of the following is NOT a polysaccharide?

   A. Cellulose
   B. Fat
   C. Glycogen
   D. Starch

43. Pinocytosis is a phenomenon which involves which one of the following?

   A. Ciliary action
   B. Annual ring differentiation
   C. Centrosome division
   D. Cellular ingestion

44. In mitosis, chromatids may first be observed during which one of the following?

   A. Prophase
   B. Metaphase
   C. Anaphase
   D. Telephase

45. Usually when a bacteriophage attacks a bacterium, it injects a thread of

   A. NRA   B. ATP   C. DNA   D. FSH

46. Which one of the following was the first protein to be completely analyzed?

   A. Albumin   B. Thyroxin   C. Insulin   D. Casein

47. One kind of crop that should NOT be planted on a hillside is

   A. alfalfa   B. corn   C. timothy   D. vetch

48. Of the following, the plants that grow best in shady environments are

   A. bur-reeds
   B. cattails
   C. ferns
   D. goldenrods

49. The genus to which the largest conifers in the United States belong is

    A. Pinus
    B. Quercus
    C. Ulmus
    D. Sequoia

50. An example of a plant that has its seeds dispersed chiefly by animals is which one of the following?

    A. Ash
    B. Burdock
    C. Maple
    D. Thistle

KEY (CORRECT ANSWERS)

1. D	11. D	21. C	31. D	41. C
2. B	12. C	22. B	32. C	42. B
3. D	13. C	23. B	33. B	43. D
4. D	14. D	24. C	34. C	44. A
5. C	15. A	25. C	35. A	45. C
6. A	16. B	26. B	36. A	46. C
7. B	17. B	27. B	37. C	47. B
8. A	18. A	28. B	38. A	48. C
9. A	19. C	29. A	39. C	49. D
10. C	20. D	30. B	40. D	50. B

EXAMINATION SECTION
TEST 1

DIRECTIONS: Each question or incomplete statement is followed by several suggested answers or completions. Select the one that BEST answers the question or completes the statement. *PRINT THE LETTER OF THE CORRECT ANSWER IN THE SPACE AT THE RIGHT.*

1. Phagocytosis is aided by the presence of

    A. lysins
    B. opsonins
    C. antitoxins
    D. precipitins

2. Thyroid tumors MAY be diagnosed with the aid of radioactive

    A. carbon
    B. sodium
    C. phosphorus
    D. iodine

3. Heparin is used as a(n)

    A. anticonvulsive
    B. depressant
    C. stimulant
    D. anticoagulant

4. The Haversian canals are located in

    A. skeletal muscle
    B. nerve centers
    C. bones
    D. glands

5. A PRIMARY difference between RNA and DNA is that the former

    A. contains uracil
    B. lacks adenine
    C. contains thymine
    D. contains fewer oxygen atoms

6. Sex-linked genes were FIRST discovered by

    A. Morgan
    B. Dobzhansky
    C. Castle
    D. Muller

7. Which one of the following terms involves ALL the others?

    A. Stock   B. Graft   C. Scion   D. Cambium

8. The Russian geneticist who stressed the role of inheritance in crop plants is

    A. Dobzhansky
    B. Vavilov
    C. Lysenko
    D. Karpechenko

9. In the mammal, fertilization USUALLY occurs in the

    A. uterine (Fallopian) tubes
    B. ovaries
    C. body of the uterus
    D. cervix of the uterus

10. A color-blind father will MOST probably transmit the gene for colorblindness to

    A. 50% of his sons
    B. 50% of his grandsons
    C. 100% of his sons
    D. 100% of his daughters

11. Gynandromorphs appear in Drosophila because of

    A. cytoplasmic inheritance
    B. autosomes
    C. loss of X chromosome
    D. gain of Y chromosome

12. In which one of the following were giant chromosomes discovered?

    A. Fruit fly
    B. Man
    C. Garden pea
    D. Four o'clock

13. Since the ability to taste phenylthiocarbide is a dominant trait among humans, if both parents are non-tasters, the percent of children LIKELY to be tasters is

    A. zero B. 25 C. 50 D. 75

14. Cranial capacity is a measurement of

    A. intelligence
    B. cephalic index
    C. internal volume of the brain case
    D. the size of the cerebellum

15. Hereditary variations in plants have been produced by which one of the following?

    A. Auxins
    B. Colchicine
    C. 2, 4-D
    D. Gibberellins

16. Heteroecious can BEST be described as pertaining to a

    A. parasite requiring two hosts for completion of its life cycle
    B. form producing both kinds of gametes in the same individual
    C. plant where self-pollination is common
    D. plant producing two kinds of spores that develop into two kinds of gametophytes

17. Fossil imprints are MOST likely to be found in which one of the following?

    A. Granite B. Lava C. Marble D. Shale

18. Of the following, which organism is STILL in existence?

    A. Tyrannosaurus
    B. Equus
    C. Cynodont
    D. Trilobite

19. Of the following, the MOST common reason why an organism introduced into a new area often thrives there is the

    A. *presence* of a green plant
    B. *presence* of a plentiful food supply
    C. *presence* of competitors
    D. *absence* of its natural enemies

20. Of the following, the factor in the environment NOT affected by the destruction of eel-grass in shallow coastal waters is the

   A. number of scallops and mussels
   B. number of migratory ducks
   C. salinity of the water
   D. depth of mud in mud flats

21. Plants which live in desert regions are called

   A. hydrophytes   B. xerophytes
   C. mesophytes   D. halophytes

22. Which one of the following is an alga found growing on the north side of tree trunks?

   A. Protococcus   B. Pandorina
   C. Volvox   D. Ulothrix

23. Which one of the following is illustrated by the growth of desert plants in the Southwest? _____ community

   A. Climax   B. Pioneer   C. Symbiotic   D. Independent

24. To which one of the following can the survival of flowering plants BEST be attributed?

   A. Absence of a vascular system
   B. Development of the fruit
   C. Development of an extensive root system
   D. Ability to carry on vegetative propagation

25. A manner in which organic compounds might have been produced ORIGINALLY on the earth was demonstrated by

   A. Miller   B. Oparin   C. Palade   D. Stanley

26. Elastic tissue is of the type known as

   A. connective   B. muscular
   C. nerve   D. epithelial

27. Of the following terms, the one that includes ALL the others is

   A. gametogenesis   B. oogenesis
   C. spermatogenesis   D. reduction division

28. Cutting away a complete ring of bark from a tree stops the passage of material through the

   A. medullary rays   B. xylem
   C. phloem   D. tracheics

29. Independent assortment does NOT always occur in hihybrid crosses. This may be the result of

   A. recessiveness   B. linkage
   C. segregation   D. dominance

30. An example of a pair of homologous structures is the

   A. wing of a housefly and the wing of a bat
   B. front leg of a cat and the wing of a bird
   C. flipper of a whale and the tail of a fish
   D. trunk of a tree and the trunk of an elephant

31. The relation between clover plants and nitrogen-fixing bacteria is a form of

   A. parasitism   B. commensalism
   C. saprophytism   D. symbiosis

32. Autumnal abscission of leaves benefits deciduous trees PRIMARILY in

   A. conserving water   B. eliminating waste products
   C. slowing respiration   D. allowing the tree to rest

33. A wire clothesline was tied six feet from the ground around an 18' elm tree. When the tree grew to a height of 36', the height, in feet, of the line above the ground was

   A. 6   B. 9   C. 12   D. 18

34. The portions of the solar spectrum MOST effective as a source of energy for photosynthesis are the

   A. yellow and blue   B. green and blue
   C. red and violet   D. indigo and green

35. The role of chlorophyll in photosynthesis is similar to the role of

   A. an enzyme in digestion
   B. glucose in respiration
   C. bile in fat digestion
   D. carbon dioxide in respiration

36. In a given sample of blood, clumping occurred with both A serum and B serum. The blood type was

   A. A   B. B   C. AB   D. O

37. Blood plasma from which the fibrinogen has been removed is known as

   A. blood concentrate   B. serum
   C. antibody component   D. hormone complement

38. A type of blood bank from which reserves of red blood corpuscles may be quickly mobilized when needed by the body is the

   A. intestinal mesentery B. liver
   C. bone marrow   D. spleen

39. The LOWEST concentration of nitrogenous waste GENERALLY may be found in blood passing through the

   A. pulmonary artery   B. hepatic vein
   C. renal artery   D. renal vein

40. A drastic type of anemia, erythroblastosis fetalis, is caused by

    A. a deficiency of iron in the diet
    B. virus invasion of red blood corpuscles
    C. antibodies induced in the pregnant mother by fetal antigens
    D. a fetus that is Rh negative

41. Pleurococcus may MOST often be found

    A. on the moist shaded side of a tree trunk
    B. on the surface of a still pond
    C. under a rock
    D. in a running stream

42. The movement of raw materials and carbohydrates from one region to another within a plant is known as

    A. translocation
    B. transpiration
    C. transmutation
    D. transfusion

43. Oxygen enters the blood because

    A. there is a higher partial pressure of O_2 in the lungs
    B. there is a higher partial pressure of CO_2 in the lungs
    C. blood contains hemoglobin
    D. there is a higher partial pressure of O_2 in the blood

44. Failure to blood to clot readily when exposed to air MAY be due to a(n)

    A. oversupply of erythrocytes
    B. deficiency of leucocytes
    C. overabundance of fibrin
    D. inadequacy of thrombokinase

45. Acetylsalicylic acid retards the clotting of blood. This would be ADVANTAGEOUS in

    A. cancer
    B. coronary thrombosis
    C. hemorrhage of the lungs
    D. an appendectomy

46. Failure of lymph to circulate would MOST directly affect

    A. fat digestion
    B. transport between the body cells and blood
    C. production of red blood cells
    D. circulation of blood platelets

47. The respiratory blood pigment found in mollusks is

    A. hemoglobin
    B. hemocyanin
    C. hemerythrin
    D. chlorocruorin

48. A rabbit sensitized to human blood gives the precipitin-clumping reaction LEAST promptly when its serum is added to the whole blood of a

    A. lemur   B. human   C. gorilla   D. chimpanzee

49. The chemicals that cause clumping of the erythrocytes in the blood are found in

    A. platelets
    B. red corpuscles
    C. white corpuscles
    D. plasma

50. In the human fetus, blood flows directly between the left and right auricles. This would indicate that

    A. the pulmonary system does not function before birth
    B. the heart does not function before birth
    C. the heart of the fetus carries only unoxygenated blood
    D. only the ventricles of the fetal heart are functional before birth

KEY (CORRECT ANSWERS)

1. B	11. C	21. B	31. D	41. A
2. D	12. A	22. A	32. A	42. A
3. D	13. A	23. A	33. A	43. A
4. C	14. C	24. B	34. C	44. D
5. A	15. B	25. A	35. A	45. B
6. A	16. A	26. A	36. C	46. B
7. B	17. D	27. A	37. B	47. B
8. C	18. B	28. C	38. D	48. A
9. A	19. D	29. B	39. D	49. D
10. D	20. C	30. B	40. C	50. A

TEST 2

DIRECTIONS: Each question or incomplete statement is followed by several suggested answers or completions. Select the one that BEST answers the question or completes the statement. *PRINT THE LETTER OF THE CORRECT ANSWER IN THE SPACE AT THE RIGHT.*

1. Sap rises in woody stems because of root pressure and   1.____

    A. transpiration pull   B. enzyme action
    C. photosynthesis   D. molecular adhesion

2. Vascular plants contain vessels called xylem and   2.____

    A. cambium   B. phloem
    C. meristem   D. lenticels

3. The SPECIFIC function of light energy in the process of photosynthesis is to   3.____

    A. activate chlorophyll   B. split water
    C. reduce carbon dioxide   D. synthesize glucose

4. Stored food for the embryo of a bean seed is found in the   4.____

    A. testa   B. plumule   C. cotyledons   D. hypocotyl

5. Of the following, an example of carnivorous plants is the   5.____

    A. sundew   B. mandrake   C. cowslip   D. jewelweed

6. In the structure of a flower, the stigma is MOST closely associated with the   6.____

    A. style   B. pistil   C. sepal   D. ovule

7. Of the following animal phyla, the one which is PROBABLY more varied and abundant   7.____
   now than in previous geological periods is the

    A. Protozoa   B. Bryozoa
    C. Brachiopoda   D. Echinodermata

8. Of the following, one difference between frog and man is that the frog has NO   8.____

    A. salivary glands   B. thyroid gland
    C. pancreas   D. adrenal gland

9. Of the following organisms, the one that is NOT in the same taxonomic class as the oth-   9.____
   ers is the

    A. salamander   B. mud puppy
    C. newt   D. lizard

10. The vocal organ of birds is the   10.____

     A. trachea   B. larynx   C. syrinx   D. air sac

11. Of the following, the marsupial native to the United States is the   11.____

     A. raccoon   B. wombat   C. opossum   D. armadillo

205

12. Of the following, a structure found in mammals but NOT in reptiles is the

    A. lung   B. brain   C. diaphragm   D. ventricle

13. The FIRST fully terrestrial vertebrates were the

    A. amphibia   B. reptiles   C. birds   D. mammals

14. A cartilaginous vertebrate that parasitizes fish is the

    A. pilot fish   B. lamprey
    C. moray eel   D. barracuda

15. Of the following, the one to which the horseshoe crab is MOST closely related is the

    A. blue crab   B. lobster
    C. garden spider   D. chambered nautilus

16. The titanotheres were a group of fossil

    A. fish   B. amphibians   C. reptiles   D. mammals

17. Of the following, a crustacean that lives on land is the

    A. centipede   B. millipede   C. sow bug   D. tick

18. Of the following, the one that is NOT an animal is the

    A. sea lily   B. sea cucumber
    C. sand dollar   D. diatom

19. Of the following, the hydra is MOST closely related to the

    A. coral   B. roundworm   C. flatworm   D. sponge

20. A PROBABLY unforeseen result of the widespread use of DDT is the

    A. control of mosquitoes
    B. development of insects immune to DDT
    C. development of fish immune to DDT
    D. destruction of harmful birds

21. Oxygen enters protozoa CHIEFLY through the

    A. surface protoplasm   B. vacuoles
    C. oral grooves   D. pseudopodia

22. Air passes into and out of the insect body by way of

    A. skin   B. lungs   C. gills   D. tracheae

23. The BEST basis for choosing a bull to sire a productive dairy herd is

    A. milk production by the bull's female ancestors
    B. milk production by the bull's sisters
    C. milk production by the bull's daughters
    D. the physical characteristics of the bull itself

24. The result of the loss of a retina in an eye is

    A. nearsightedness
    B. farsightedness
    C. astigmatism
    D. lack of vision in the affected eye

25. The LARGEST percentage of the salt excreted from the body normally passes out through the

    A. kidneys
    B. skin
    C. lachrymal glands
    D. large intestine

26. A lack of which one of the following vitamins causes polyneuritis?

    A. Choline B. Niacin C. Riboflavin D. Thiamin

27. Myelinated nerve fibers are USUALLY involved in the performance of the

    A. autonomic reflexes
    B. secretions
    C. skeletal muscles
    D. smooth muscles

28. Balance and muscular coordination are LARGELY controlled by the

    A. cerebellum
    B. cerebrum
    C. frontal lobe
    D. occipital lobe

29. The sciatic nerve is associated with contractions of the muscles in the

    A. arm B. leg C. neck D. shoulder

30. Of the following, the one which is an example of an epiphyte is

    A. clover B. orchid C. dodder D. Indian pipe

31. Hormones extracted from some plants that can induce earlier blooming in other plants are known as

    A. chromogens
    B. aerogens
    C. anthogens
    D. zymogens

32. A fleshy receptacle is the MAIN edible portion of which one of the following?

    A. Pear
    B. Orange
    C. Raspberry
    D. Watermelon

33. The structure in a flower that is homologous to the prothallus of a fern is the

    A. anther
    B. embryo sac
    C. ovary
    D. spore mother cell

34. The cambium layer in a plant serves which one of the following purposes?

    A. To protect the plant
    B. To support the plant
    C. As a food storage organ
    D. To produce new cells

35. Which one of the following is TRUE of root hair cells?

    A. Consist of a single cell
    B. Derived from xylem
    C. Undergo rapid cell division
    D. Become multinucleated

36. Plant turgor is DIRECTLY affected by the contents of the cell structures called the

    A. microsomes
    B. mitochondria
    C. vacuoles
    D. plasmosomes

37. Stomates can BEST be demonstrated with which one of the following?

    A. Raw potatoes
    B. Elodea leaves
    C. Fern fronds
    D. Lettuce leaves

38. Which one of the following is a characteristic of the monocotyledons?

    A. Netted veined leaves
    B. Annual rings
    C. Seeds with two masses of stored food
    D. Conducting tissue in distinct bundles

39. The bark of trees is composed of cells derived from which one of the following pairs?

    A. Xylem and pith
    B. Xylem and cambium
    C. Phloem and bast
    D. Phloem and xylem

40. Sunken protected stomates would MOST likely be found on

    A. hydrophytes
    B. mesophytes
    C. saprophytes
    D. xerophytes

41. In a bean seed, all of the following parts belong to the new sporophyte generation EXCEPT

    A. cotyledon
    B. hypocotyl
    C. plumule
    D. testa

42. Meiosis occurs in the part of the flower called the

    A. anther   B. calyx   C. corolla   D. stigma

43. Pioneer experiments in photosynthesis were performed by which one of the following?

    A. Ingen-Housz
    B. Pasteur
    C. Redi
    D. Nordenskjold

44. What part of a seed plant is homologous to the spore of a fern?

    A. Embryo   B. Ovule   C. Pollen   D. Seed

45. A tissue which is NORMALLY triploid is found in the seed of which one of the following?

    A. Bean   B. Corn   C. Pea   D. Peach

46. A large locule can be readily demonstrated in which one of the following?

    A. Apple   B. Orange   C. Peach   D. Pear

47. A beech-maple forest would MOST likely be found in which one of the following? 47._____

    A. Adirondack Mountains   B. Great Plains
    C. Mississippi delta   D. Rocky Mountains

48. De Vries discovered his FIRST mutants in the flower called 48._____

    A. sweet pea   B. peanut   C. petunia   D. primrose

49. Mutualism is BEST shown in which one of the following? 49._____

    A. Proifera   B. Slime molds
    C. Viruses   D. Lichens

50. To help replenish the supply of nitrogen compounds in the soil, the planting of corn should be rotated with that of which one of the following? 50._____

    A. Rye   B. Alfalfa   C. Oats   D. Barley

KEY (CORRECT ANSWERS)

1. A	11. C	21. A	31. C	41. D
2. B	12. C	22. D	32. A	42. A
3. A	13. B	23. C	33. B	43. A
4. C	14. B	24. D	34. D	44. C
5. A	15. C	25. A	35. A	45. B
6. A	16. D	26. D	36. C	46. B
7. A	17. C	27. C	37. D	47. A
8. A	18. D	28. A	38. D	48. D
9. D	19. A	29. B	39. C	49. D
10. C	20. B	30. B	40. D	50. B

TEST 3

DIRECTIONS: Each question or incomplete statement is followed by several suggested answers or completions. Select the one that BEST answers the question or completes the statement. *PRINT THE LETTER OF THE CORRECT ANSWER IN THE SPACE AT THE RIGHT.*

1. Of the following, the one which is an organ of equilibrium found in some invertebrates is the 1.____

   A. labyrinth
   B. cochlea
   C. semicircular canal
   D. statocyst

2. Muscular contractions known as tetany result from an undersecretion of the 2.____

   A. thyroid
   B. parathyroid
   C. adrenals
   D. thymus

3. Organelles which serve as receptors in unicellular organisms are which one of the following? 3.____

   A. Myonemes
   B. Chromatophores
   C. Flagella
   D. Neurofibrils

4. The transmission of impulses across synapses and myoneural junctions of the autonomic system depends on neuro-humors such as 4.____

   A. acetylcholine
   B. actomyosin
   C. atropine
   D. avidin

5. An eye is a light receptor in which the 5.____

   A. rods distinguish color
   B. visual purple is formed in the vitreous humor
   C. blind spot contains only cones
   D. fovea centralis has the most acute vision

6. Protista is a term that is used to include ONLY 6.____

   A. one-celled animals
   B. unicellular plants
   C. acellular organisms
   D. multicellular organisms

7. In the nitrogen cycle, the bacteria which change proteins to ammonia are known as 7.____

   A. bacteria of decay
   B. denitrifying bacteria
   C. nitrite bacteria
   D. nitrogen-fixing bacteria

8. True motility is present in bacteria that possess which one of the following? 8.____

   A. Cilia   B. Pseudopods   C. Flagella   D. Cirri

9. Bacteria of decay may change dead leaves into which one of the following? 9.____

   A. Green manure
   B. Humus
   C. Loam
   D. Fungi

10. Of the following, a disinfectant that liberates chlorine is 10.____

    A. Dakin's solution
    B. hydrogen peroxide
    C. tricresol
    D. merthiolate

210

11. During the development of a starfish embryo, the process of invagination results in forming the stage called the

    A. blastula   B. gastrula   C. morula   D. neurula

12. Which one of the following mammalian arteries is homologous to the third aortic arch of fish?

    A. Cerebral   B. Carotid
    C. Innominate   D. Mandibular

13. In the frog, the oxygenated and deoxygenated blood entering the ventricle are kept separated by the

    A. interventricular septum
    B. auricular-ventricular valve
    C. angle at which the blood reflects from the ventricular wall
    D. alternate pulsations of the muscles of the ventricular wall

14. The secretory mantle is a distinguishing feature of which one of the following?

    A. Echinodermata   B. Bryozoa
    C. Mollusca   D. Protochordata

15. Among land vertebrates, internal fertilization is the rule because of the adaptive characteristics of the

    A. oviduct   B. sperm   C. uterus   D. vas deferens

16. Recently, a *screw-worm* pest has been eliminated from the southeastern part of the United States by means of

    A. DDT   B. 2-4D
    C. natural enemies D. irradiation of males

17. A structure in chick embryos that forms outside of the body and later becomes enclosed is the

    A. heart   B. lens   C. liver   D. stomach

18. Peripatus has nephridial tubes and tracheal tubes and is, therefore, considered to be an intermediate between annelids and

    A. anthropods   B. bryozoa
    C. mollusks   D. platyhelminthes

19. A mesodermal structure that gradually disappears as bones form around it is the

    A. cervical arch   B. epiglottis
    C. notochord   D. sigmoid flexure

20. Internal fertilization and external development are ALWAYS the natural course of reproduction in which one of the following?

    A. Aves   B. Ophidia   C. Pisces   D. Reptilia

21. An epididymus is present in the reproductive systems of male 21.____

    A. lizards B. mice C. toads D. tuna

22. Which one of the following is found in mammals but NOT in other vertebrates? 22.____

    A. Clavicle B. Nephrostome
    C. Adrenal gland D. Diaphragm

23. Which one of the following purposes is achieved by the pebbles in the gizzards of chickens? 23.____

    A. Slow the absorption of nutrients
    B. Stimulate peristalsis in the intestines
    C. Help in the mastication of food
    D. Supply minerals for egg shell formation

24. A heart with a single auricle and a single ventricle is characteristic of adult 24.____

    A. amphibians B. arthropods
    C. birds D. fish

25. The corpora allata are small glandular organs found in which one of the following? 25.____

    A. Moths B. Crayfish C. Mammals D. Salamanders

26. The microscopic structure in a flower that contains the egg cell is the 26.____

    A. anther B. embryo sac
    C. locule D. microgametophyte

27. The structure in the corn seed that functions in the same way as does the cotyledon in a bean seed is the 27.____

    A. epicotyl B. endosperm C. pericarp D. plumule

28. The fleshy, edible part of an apple is derived MAINLY from the part of the flower called the 28.____

    A. pericarp B. pistil C. receptacle D. sepal

29. The placenta of a mammal is biologically MOST important because it 29.____

    A. is heavily vascularized and affords large surface area for interchange between separate vascular systems
    B. supports the foetus in a nourishing fluid
    C. protects the embryo from mechanical injury
    D. is a passageway for direct arterial connection from mother into the foetus

30. Of the following vertebrates, the one in which reproduction is characterized by internal fertilization of the ovum and external development of the embryo is the 30.____

    A. pigeon B. guppy C. rabbit D. whale

31. The Graafan follicle

   A. supports sebaceous glands necessary for keeping the skin soft
   B. produces the ovum during the menstrual cycle
   C. secretes the hormone secretin
   D. stimulates the development of secondary sex characteristics in males

32. The process that takes place on or about the 14th day of the menstrual cycle in humans is

   A. the breakdown of the uterus lining
   B. denigration
   C. ovulation
   D. parturition

33. In a breed of chickens that has 3 distinct color in plumage (white, tan, brown), if 2 tan birds are bred, the offspring would be

   A. all tan
   B. 50% tan, 50% brown
   C. 25% tan, 50% brown, 25% white
   D. 25% brown, 50% tan, 25% white

34. If a tall, red-flowered pea plant (TtRr) is crossed with a tall, whiteflowered pea plant (TTrr), the percentage of offspring that would be tall and white-flowered would be

   A. 25   B. 50   C. 75   D. 100

35. T.H. Morgan and his co-workers were the FIRST to offer experimental proof that

   A. during formation of gametes there is separation of maternal and paternal factors
   B. genes are located on chromosomes in a linear arrangement
   C. a single phenotype may be the result of more than one gene
   D. non-allelomorphic factors segregate independently

36. Desoxyribose nucleic acid (DNA) is believed to be the MOST important constituent of

   A. centrioles   B. centrosomes
   C. chromosomes   D. Golgi bodies

37. The Nobel Prize winner who demonstrated that genes can be caused to mutate by x-rays is

   A. Correns   B. Dunn   C. Muller   D. Sturtevant

38. Of the following, the fossil of the MOST recent primate is called the

   A. Homo Neanderthalensis   B. Homarus Americanus
   C. Plasianthropus   D. Pithecanthropus

39. In an unfolded cliff of stratified rock, the sequence of fossils from the bottom up would be expected to be

   A. mastodon, trilobite, archaeornis, Brontosaurus
   B. trilobite, Brontosaurus, archaeornis, mammoth

C. Allosaurus, ammonite, Hesperornis, Homo
D. ammonite, Hesperornis, trilobite, Sinanthropus

40. An animal with a water-vascular system, tube feet, and a spiny skin would belong to the phylum

    A. echinodermata B. annelida
    C. molluscoidea   D. platyhelminthea

41. The organism that causes the disease trichinosis is a member of the phylum that includes

    A. annelids   B. flatworms   C. roundworms   D. fungi

42. Antheridia and archegonia are reproductive organs found in

    A. Angiosperms   B. Basidiomycetes
    C. Bryophytes   D. Schizophytes

43. The gametophyte generation is dominant in

    A. ferns   B. grains   C. legumes   D. mosses

44. The structures that transport water up the stem of woody plants are the

    A. bast fibers   B. parenchyma cells
    C. sieve tubes   D. tracheids

45. When the bark is stripped from a tree, the vital vascular tissue removed is the

    A. phloem   B. cork cambium
    C. pith   D. vessels

46. Protein synthesis by green plants involves the combination of carbohydrate products with

    A. fats   B. minerals   C. steroids   D. vitamins

47. The cells in the chlorenchyma adapted to perform photosynthesis are called

    A. companion   B. fibrovascular
    C. palisade   D. pith

48. Examination of soils in some areas have shown that what is now basswood and maple forestland was once occupied by lakes. The lake first choked up with water plants, and swamp vegetation appeared. Then, spruce and pine grew. Finally, maple and basswood became the dominant form. The above process is BEST known as

    A. ecological succession   B. geological evidence
    C. natural selection   D. survival of the fittest

49. An insect that destroys a large number of plant lice is the

    A. hawkmoth   B. ichneumon fly
    C. ladybird beetle (ladybug)   D. robber fly

50. The Papanicolaou (PAP) test is used to discover early cases of

    A. cancer   B. typhoid
    C. tuberculosis   D. syphilis

KEY (CORRECT ANSWERS)

1. D	11. B	21. B	31. B	41. C
2. B	12. B	22. D	32. C	42. C
3. B	13. C	23. C	33. D	43. D
4. A	14. C	24. D	34. B	44. D
5. D	15. B	25. A	35. B	45. A
6. C	16. D	26. B	36. C	46. B
7. A	17. A	27. B	37. C	47. C
8. C	18. A	28. C	38. A	48. A
9. B	19. C	29. A	39. B	49. C
10. A	20. A	30. A	40. A	50. A

TEST 4

DIRECTIONS: Each question or incomplete statement is followed by several suggested answers or completions. Select the one that BEST answers the question or completes the statement. *PRINT THE LETTER OF THE CORRECT ANSWER IN THE SPACE AT THE RIGHT.*

1. The following vitamins are members of the B complex, with the exception of

    A. riboflavin
    B. pantothenic acid
    C. inositol
    D. tocopherol

    1._____

2. Of the following, the blood cells which are NOT manufactured in the red bone marrow are the

    A. lymphocytes
    B. granulocytes
    C. red blood cells
    D. blood platelets

    2._____

3. The air we inhale when we take a deep breath is called _____ air.

    A. tidal
    B. supplemental
    C. complemental
    D. residual

    3._____

4. The liver is an organ which

    A. receives blood from the hepatic vein
    B. produces the enzyme erepsin
    C. contains Kupffer cells that absorb fat globules
    D. carries on diapedesis

    4._____

5. Which one of the following statements does NOT apply to enzymes? They

    A. are all made of an apoenzyme and a coenzyme
    B. are usually not specific in their effect
    C. lose their stability at high temperature
    D. can function outside of living cells

    5._____

6. The digestive hormone that stimulates the emptying of the gall bladder is

    A. cholecystokinin
    B. pancreatin
    C. enterogastrone
    D. gastrin

    6._____

7. A systolic blood pressure normal for a high school boy would be CLOSEST to which one of the following?

    A. 100
    B. 125
    C. 150
    D. 175

    7._____

8. Which one of the following does NOT describe a phase of blood clotting?

    A. Vitamin K is involved in prothrombin formation by the liver.
    B. Thrombokinase is released by blood platelets after an injury.
    C. Prothrombin combines with thrombokinase and sodium ions to form thrombin.
    D. Thrombin unites with fibrinogen to form fibrin.

    8._____

9. In vertebrates, blood cells which carry oxygen are known as

   A. leucocytes B. erythrocytes
   C. thrombocytes D. monocytes

10. The suction-tension theory seems to explain

    A. transpiration in plants
    B. transport of water by plants
    C. movement of nutrients in phloem
    D. cohesion of water molecules in xylem

11. During its development, the cat embryo obtains its food through the

    A. yolk sac B. placenta C. ova D. albumen

12. Abiogenesis can BEST be described as

    A. gamete formation B. asexual reproduction
    C. evolution D. spontaneous generation

13. Alternation of generation in plants refers to the

    A. alternation of diploid and haploid generations
    B. alternation of mature and immature forms
    C. alternation of apospory and apogamy
    D. seasonal growth cycle

14. Meiosis occurs during the

    A. abnormal division of cancer cells
    B. animal cell division
    C. plant cell division
    D. formation of haploid cells

15. The development of unfertilized daphnia eggs is an example of

    A. maturation B. metamorphosis
    C. parthenogenesis D. ontogeny

16. Which one of the following pairs is NOT correctly matched?

    A. Dandelion - parachute B. Touch-me-not - barbs
    C. Maple - wings D. Burdock - hooks

17. Which one of the following is NOT a fruit?

    A. Potato B. Tomato
    C. Cucumber D. Green pepper

18. Of the following, the plants which reproduce by means of spores are

    A. carrots B. grasses
    C. fruit trees D. ferns

19. Which one of the following causes tobacco mosaic?

    A. Mineral deficiencies B. Radiation
    C. Bacteria D. Viruses

20. Dichlorophenolindophenol is used to test for

    A. vitamin C
    B. amino acids
    C. polysaccharides
    D. vitamin A

21. Which of the following is NOT an example of a modified stem?

    A. Spines in the cactus
    B. Thorns in the honey locust
    C. Runners in the strawberry
    D. Adventitious roots in the poison ivy

22. The young stem of a dicotyledonous plant has

    A. scattered fibrovascular bundles
    B. no cambium between xylem and phloem
    C. a central core of pith
    D. medullary rays around the cortex

23. The sella turcica contains the

    A. pituitary gland
    B. lobules of the liver
    C. renal papillae
    D. fetal villi

24. The thickness of the specimen which may be seen in focus at one time is referred to as

    A. magnification
    B. resolution
    C. depth of focus
    D. definition

25. The experiments of Avery, MacLeod, and McCarty proved conclusively that

    A. transduction occurs in bacteria
    B. DNA molecules are arranged in a double helix
    C. sickle-cell anemia is caused by a mutant gene
    D. DNA carries genetic information

26. In order to keep the soil of a terrarium from souring, it is ADVISABLE to add

    A. a large quantity of water
    B. charcoal
    C. only potting soil
    D. sand

27. The MOST frequent cause of cloudy water and polluted aquaria is

    A. dirty gravel
    B. diseased plants
    C. over-feeding
    D. sick fish

28. Materials can be exchanged readily through the walls of

    A. arteries and capillaries
    B. arteries and veins
    C. capillaries alone
    D. veins and capillaries

29. Cell bodies of sensory neurons lie in the

    A. blind spot
    B. dorsal root
    C. frontal lobe
    D. ventral root

30. The autonomic nervous system controls 30.____

    A. blood pressure   B. peristalsis
    C. sweating   D. all of the above

31. A muscle fiber contracts 31.____

    A. either maximally or not at all
    B. in proportion to the innervation
    C. in relation to the contraction of other muscle fibers
    D. only when ATP has been excreted

32. The rate of respiration is controlled by the 32.____

    A. decrease of oxygen in the bloodstream
    B. respiratory center in the medulla
    C. motor area in the cerebral cortex
    D. inhibiting action of the phrenic nerve

33. The glomerulus is a functioning unit in the 33.____

    A. kidney   B. skin   C. lung   D. liver

34. Amebae accomplish ingestion by means of 34.____

    A. chelipeds   B. oral grooves
    C. pseudopods   D. tentacles

35. Auxin is to the plant as one of the following is to the animal: 35.____

    A. Pepsin   B. Ptyalin   C. Rennin   D. Thyroxin

36. To kill all bacteria in milk, it is necessary to 36.____

    A. dialyze   B. sterilize
    C. pasteurize   D. homogenize

37. Peristalsis is MOST characteristic of the 37.____

    A. arteries   B. intestines   C. kidneys   D. liver

38. The energy release in the body depends upon enzyme systems which store energy in the form of the high energy bonds of 38.____

    A. ACTH   B. ATP   C. DDT   D. 2, 4D

39. There is no flow of blood from the aorta back into the heart because of the action of the _____ valve(s). 39.____

    A. bicuspid   B. mitral
    C. semi-lunar   D. tricuspid

40. The incorporation of amino acids into body protoplasm is termed 40.____

    A. absorption   B. assimilation
    C. deamination   D. digestion

41. ACTH, used in the treatment of arthritis, is derived from the

    A. adrenal   B. pancreas   C. pituitary   D. thyroid

42. Of the following materials, the one NOT classified as an antibiotic is

    A. aureomycin   B. V-penicillin
    C. terramycin   D. chromatin

43. Immediate immunity for a child exposed to diphtheria can be provided by

    A. antitoxin   B. toxin
    C. toxin-antitoxin   D. toxoid

44. Of the following, the ONLY living disease agents that have been crystallized are the

    A. proteins   B. rickettsiae
    C. spirochetes   D. viruses

45. In the following sequence, the one CORRECT sequence is

    A. cleavage, fertilization, gastrulation, metamorphosis, larva
    B. cleavage, fertilization, metamorphosis, gastrulation, larva
    C. fertilization, cleavage, gastrulation, larva, metamorphosis
    D. fertilization, gastrulation, cleavage, larva, metamorphosis

46. To distinguish a heterozygous black guinea pig from a homozygous black one,

    A. examine its physical features carefully
    B. mate it with a heterozygous black
    C. mate it with a homozygous black
    D. mate it with a white

47. A 9:3:3:1 ratio is obtained in a _____ cross involving _____ dominance.

    A. dihybrid; complete   B. dihybrid; incomplete
    C. monohybrid; complete   D. monohybrid; incomplete

48. Three of the following terms are properly grouped together. The one which does NOT belong is

    A. allantois   B. amnion   C. chorion   D. fovea

49. All genes lying on the same chromosome are said to be

    A. crossed over   B. independently assorted
    C. linked   D. segregated

50. Of the following scientists, three are associated with the same type of inquiry. The scientist who does NOT belong in the group is

    A. Darwin   B. Lamarck   C. Lysenko   D. Schwann

KEY (CORRECT ANSWERS)

1. D	11. B	21. A	31. A	41. C
2. A	12. D	22. C	32. B	42. D
3. C	13. A	23. A	33. A	43. A
4. C	14. D	24. C	34. C	44. D
5. B	15. C	25. D	35. D	45. C
6. A	16. B	26. B	36. B	46. D
7. B	17. A	27. C	37. B	47. A
8. C	18. D	28. C	38. B	48. D
9. B	19. D	29. B	39. C	49. C
10. D	20. A	30. D	40. B	50. D

TEST 5

DIRECTIONS: Each question or incomplete statement is followed by several suggested answers or completions. Select the one that BEST answers the question or completes the statement. *PRINT THE LETTER OF THE CORRECT ANSWER IN THE SPACE AT THE RIGHT.*

1. Which one of the following characteristics would be LEAST likely to distinguish mammals from other vertebrates?

    A. Seven cervical vertebrae
    B. A muscular diaphragm
    C. Mammary glands
    D. Young born alive

    1.____

2. The horns of the pronghorn antelope are UNIQUE in that they are

    A. bony structures
    B. covered with a horny material
    C. hollow inside
    D. shed annually

    2.____

3. Respiratory organs found in insects are called

    A. gills
    B. book lungs
    C. lungs
    D. tracheae

    3.____

4. Of the following, the way in which arachnids resemble arthropods is that they have

    A. four pairs of walking legs
    B. no compound eyes
    C. no antennae
    D. jointed exoskeletons

    4.____

5. Which one of the following is one of the characteristics distinguishing a lizard from a salamander?

    A. Slimy body
    B. Naked skin
    C. Claws on feet
    D. Eggs laid in water

    5.____

6. The SMALLEST mammal known is a species of

    A. mole   B. shrew   C. vole   D. lemming

    6.____

7. In which one of the following groups of animals is there found a gastrovascular cavity used for both ingestion and egestion?

    A. Protozoa and sponges
    B. Sponges and hydroids
    C. Coelenterates and flatworms
    D. Flatworms and annelids

    7.____

8. An open-type blood circulation is found in all of the following EXCEPT the

    A. earthworms   B. insects   C. Crustacea   D. mollusks

    8.____

222

9. The excretory organs of insects are called

   A. green glands
   B. nephridia
   C. Malpighian tubules
   D. glomeruli

10. Intracellular digestion occurs EXCLUSIVELY in which one of the following?

    A. Molds
    B. Sponges
    C. Carnivorous plants
    D. Echinoderms

11. The osmotic effect of water in the paramecium is controlled by the

    A. cell membrane
    B. pellicle
    C. macronucleus
    D. contractile vacuoles

12. Which one of the following is used as a mold inhibitor in the preparation of a Drosophila culture medium?

    A. Ninhydrin   B. Nipagen   C. Pyridoxin   D. Glycine

13. Which one of the following is arranged in a CORRECT sequence?

    A. Family, genus, phylum, order
    B. Order, family, species, variety
    C. Phylum, order, genus, family
    D. Kingdom, order, species, genus

14. Which one of the following represents a monocotyledonous family of plants?

    A. Legumes
    B. Water lilies
    C. Grasses
    D. Roses

15. Which one of the following pairs of animal groups consists of two groups belonging to the same phylum?

    A. Myriapods and leeches
    B. Slugs and earthworms
    C. Sand dollars and clams
    D. Tarantulas and barnacles

16. Which one of the following statements does NOT apply to the euglenophytes?

    A. They are partly plant-like and partly animal-like.
    B. They have active locomotion.
    C. Many carry on mixotrophic nutrition.
    D. True cell walls are usually present.

17. Which of the following developed the system of binomial nomenclature?

    A. Linnaeus   B. John Ray   C. Spemann   D. Driesch

18. Which one of the following terms includes all the others?

    A. Alga
    B. Fungus
    C. Thallophyte
    D. Slime mold

19. Photosynthetic phosphorylation means that
    A. photolysis has occurred in the light reaction
    B. CO_2 incorporation has taken place in the dark reaction
    C. ADP has been changed to ATP
    D. H_2O is split in the grana of the chloroplasts

20. The movement of materials through a cell membrane against a concentration gradient is called
    A. diffusion   B. osmosis
    C. active transport   D. Brownian movement

21. Which one of the following statements does NOT apply to aerobic metabolism?
    A. Pyruvic acid combines with two hydrogens to form lactic acid.
    B. Carbon compounds are decarboxylated.
    C. Acetic acid combines with oxalocetic acid to form citric acid.
    D. Carbon compounds are dehydrogenated.

22. Recent research with radioactive oxygen indicates that during photosynthesis
    A. all oxygen released comes from the water molecule
    B. whole water molecules are used in making carbohydrates
    C. all oxygen released comes from the carbon dioxide molecule
    D. oxygen released from a cell comes from both the CO_2 and H_2O

23. Bleeding gums is GENERALLY associated with a deficiency of
    A. thiamin   B. folic acid
    C. ascorbic acid   D. niacin

24. The energy for muscular contraction and flagella movement seems to come from
    A. oxygen in the environment
    B. ATP breakdown
    C. DNA control
    D. glycogen synthesis

25. It has been discovered in working with blood groups that
    A. type O people can serve as universal recipients
    B. cross-matching is unnecessary if people have the same blood type
    C. the agglutinogens are found in the red blood corpuscles
    D. type A is the rarest group

26. To provide immunity against diphtheria, a healthy child is inoculated with
    A. toxoid   B. toxin   C. antitoxin   D. germicide

27. The plant tissue which NORMALLY conducts food from leaves down to the roots is the
    A. pith   B. tracheid   C. phloem   D. cambium

28. Chloroplasts may be observed by means of a microscope demonstration of

    A. onion skin cells B. ameba
    C. elodea cells D. leaf epidermis cells

29. The part of the brain that controls the breathing reflex is the

    A. cerebrum B. cerebellum C. meninges D. medulla

30. In the classification of living things, proceeding from the largest grouping down to the smallest, the CORRECT order is phylum,

    A. class, order, genus, species
    B. class, order, species, genus
    C. genus, class, order, species
    D. order, class, genus, species

31. In the normal use of the microscope, light will strike the mirror and then proceed as follows:
    Slide,

    A. objective, ocular, lens of eye
    B. lens of eye, objective, ocular
    C. ocular, objective, lens of eye
    D. lens of eye, ocular, objective

32. When air is inhaled, all of the following activities take place EXCEPT the

    A. diaphragm contracts B. ribs are raised
    C. chest cavity is enlarged D. lungs contract

33. Another name for grain alcohol is _____ alcohol.

    A. wood B. methyl C. ethyl D. amyl

34. Oxyhemoglobin differs from hemoglobin in that it contains _____ oxygen.

    A. less B. more
    C. same amount of D. no

35. The NORMAL order of events in the clotting of blood is:

    A. Platelets, fibrin, fibrinogen, thrombin
    B. Platelets, thrombin, fibrinogen, fibrin
    C. Fibrinogen, fibrin, platelets, thrombin
    D. Fibrinogen, platelets, thrombin, fibrin

36. The tiny particles within the nucleus of a cell are known as

    A. centrosomes B. hypertonic salts
    C. chromatin D. parenchyma

37. Cancer cells that spread throughout the body are called

    A. phagocytes B. opsonins
    C. metastases D. lymphocytes

38. Viruses have been photographed through the use of the

   A. interferometer
   B. polariscope
   C. electron microscope
   D. spectroscope

39. The hormone which increases the rate of oxidation in the cells of the body is

   A. insulin
   B. thyroxin
   C. pituitrin
   D. progestin

40. The carbohydrate which the body cells can oxidize MOST readily is

   A. galactose
   B. fructose
   C. glucose
   D. sucrose

41. The thoracic duct is part of the

   A. lymphatic system
   B. heart
   C. appendix
   D. respiratory system

42. Maple and milkweed fruits may be used to demonstrate

   A. asexual reproduction
   B. regeneration
   C. appendix
   D. respiratory system

43. An example of a motile unicellular plant is a

   A. coccus
   B. yeast
   C. desmid
   D. diatom

44. The gland whose removal prevents metamorphosis in the frog is the

   A. thyroid
   B. adrenal
   C. pineal
   D. pancreas

45. A satisfactory source for obtaining paramecia for culturing in the laboratory is

   A. a stagnant pond
   B. a running stream
   C. tap water
   D. an underground river

46. To demonstrate enzymatic action, one could use milk and

   A. pepsin
   B. secretin
   C. rennin
   D. catalase

47. An infusion of unwashed grapes in water GENERALLY yields a satisfactory culture of

   A. hydra
   B. euglena
   C. paramecia
   D. yeast

48. To illustrate regeneration, one should use the

   A. planarian
   B. lobster
   C. cyclops
   D. paramecium

49. Parthenogenesis is the development of the embryo from a(n)

   A. fertilized egg
   B. zygote
   C. zygospore
   D. unfertilized egg

50. Of the following, the ion NOT found in Ringer's solution is the _____ ion.

   A. sodium
   B. chloride
   C. bicarbonate
   D. potassium

KEY (CORRECT ANSWERS)

1. D	11. D	21. A	31. A	41. A
2. D	12. B	22. A	32. D	42. D
3. D	13. B	23. C	33. C	43. D
4. D	14. C	24. B	34. B	44. A
5. C	15. D	25. C	35. B	45. A
6. B	16. D	26. A	36. C	46. C
7. C	17. A	27. C	37. C	47. D
8. A	18. C	28. C	38. C	48. A
9. C	19. C	29. D	39. B	49. D
10. B	20. C	30. A	40. C	50. C

EXAMINATION SECTION
TEST 1

DIRECTIONS: Each question or incomplete statement is followed by several suggested answers or completions. Select the one that BEST answers the question or completes the statement. *PRINT THE LETTER OF THE CORRECT ANSWER IN THE SPACE AT THE RIGHT.*

1. In the normal human body, an increase in the amount of glucose in the blood stimulates the production of
   - A. cortin
   - B. insulin
   - C. secretin
   - D. iodine
   - E. ptyalin

2. Exact similarity between chromosomes of the various cells within the same tissue of a plant or animal is LARGELY due to the mechanism of
   - A. segregation
   - B. meiosis
   - C. mitosis
   - D. fertilization
   - E. maturation

3. Marriages of closely related persons are USUALLY inadvisable from a biological standpoint because
   - A. undesirable recessive characters are more likely to appear in following generations
   - B. such unions are likely to be sterile
   - C. desirable characteristics, even when dominant, are less likely to be transmitted to future generations
   - D. such unions generally produce physically weaker children
   - E. at least one-fourth of the children are likely to be hemophiles

4. Much of the water entering an amoeba by osmosis is eliminated by the action of the
   - A. contractile vacuole
   - B. gastric vacuole
   - C. ectoplasm
   - D. cytoplasmic crystals
   - E. pseudopodia

5. The rate of flow (quantity per second) of man's blood is GREATEST in the
   - A. venae cavae
   - B. radial artery
   - C. portal vein
   - D. capillaries
   - E. aorta

6. MOST of the world's supply of sugar as a commercial product is obtained from _____ and _____.
   - A. leaves; stems
   - B. fruits; stems
   - C. roots; stems
   - D. seeds; stems
   - E. seeds; roots

7. The essential cellular component divided and redistributed by the process of mitosis is the
   - A. plasma membrane
   - B. cytoplasm
   - C. plastid
   - D. chromatin
   - E. central spindle

8. The discharge of adrenalin into the blood causes

   A. dilation of the blood vessels of the stomach
   B. increased absorption of sugar by the liver
   C. an increase in the speed and force of the heart beat
   D. constriction of the blood vessels of the muscles
   E. a slowing down of respiration

9. Synthesis of glucose from carbon dioxide and water in green plants occurs ONLY in the

   A. epidermis
   B. sieve tubes
   C. cambium
   D. chlorophyll-bearing cells
   E. root hairs

10. Identify the TRUE statement regarding syphilis.

    A. It is transmitted only by sexual contact.
    B. It attacks mainly the reproductive organs.
    C. Its treatment is the same as that for gonorrhea.
    D. Its transmission from one generation to the next follows Mendel's laws.
    E. It is possible to have a latent form of the disease without recognizable symptoms.

11. Similarities in the characteristics of identical twins are caused PRINCIPALLY by

    A. the presence of similar genes in all cells
    B. similar environmental conditions before birth
    C. similar environmental conditions after birth
    D. simultaneous fertilization of an ovum by two similar sperm cells
    E. identical genetic mutation

12. Gametes differ from spores in that gametes

    A. may unite and form zygotes
    B. are produced only by gametophytes
    C. are produced only by animals
    D. are capable of independent motion
    E. are always the larger in size

13. The poisonous effect on the human body of inhaled carbon monoxide is caused by its

    A. chemical action on lung tissue
    B. replacement of the oxygen in oxyhemoglobin
    C. insolubility in blood plasma
    D. forming insoluble precipitates in the blood
    E. paralyzing effect on the respiratory center of the brain

14. Tropisms of leaves are often produced DIRECTLY by

    A. turgor changes in certain cells
    B. contractions of wood fibers
    C. electrical conductivity of sieve tubes
    D. digestion of starch
    E. increase of sugar in the cells

15. A climax community is MOST likely to be found in regions where   15._____

    A. man has greatly modified his surroundings
    B. there are no dominant organisms
    C. conditions have remained relatively constant for a period of many years
    D. distinct changes in climatic conditions have recently occurred
    E. plants are relatively uniform in size

16. An internal secretion of the mucosa of the upper part of the small intestine stimulates the   16._____

    A. flow of ptyalin
    B. flow of pancreatic juices
    C. dilation of the cardiac sphincter
    D. production of thyroxin
    E. absorption of water in the large intestine

17. A hyperthyroid condition is characterized by   17._____

    A. low blood pressure
    B. a tendency toward obesity
    C. low body temperature
    D. increased metabolism
    E. severely retarded mental activity

18. Which of the following types of cells in the human male contains one-half the ordinary number of chromosomes?   18._____

    A. All of the somatic cells
    B. Somatic cell of the reproductive organs only
    C. Spermatozoa
    D. Primary spermatocytes
    E. T-Cells

Questions 19-20.

DIRECTIONS: Questions 19 and 20 are to be answered on the basis of the following information.
S = short-haired (dominant)
s = long-haired (recessive)

19. The parents of a litter of long-haired cats are   19._____

    A. SS+Ss   B. SS+ss   C. Ss+Ss
    D. Ss+ss   E. ss+ss

20. The parents of a litter of short-haired hybrid cats are MOST likely to be   20._____

    A. SS+Ss   B. SS+ss   C. Ss+Ss
    D. Ss+ss   E. SS+SS

Questions 21-23.

DIRECTIONS: Questions 21 through 23 are to be answered on the basis of the following diagram.

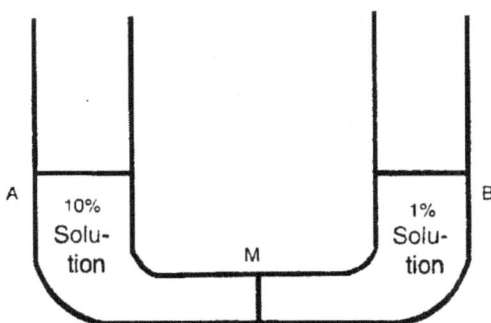

A 10% solution of cane sugar in water (A) is separated from a 1% solution of cane sugar in water (B) by a membrane (M) permeable to water but NOT to cane sugar. The levels of the two liquids are the same.

21. Molecules of water will pass through the membrane 21.___

    A. in one direction only
    B. in both directions at all times
    C. until the total number of molecules is the same on both sides
    D. only until the solution on one side is saturated
    E. only until a final constant difference in level is attained; then their passage will cease

22. When equilibrium between the two solutions is attained, 22.___

    A. the levels of the two solutions will be equal
    B. there will be an equal number of sugar molecules in each solution
    C. there will be an equal number of water molecules in each solution
    D. no molecules will pass through the membrane in either direction
    E. equal numbers of water molecules will be passing through the membrane in each direction

23. If the membrane were equally permeable to water and to sugar, 23.___

    A. the concentration in A and B would remain unchanged, even after a long period of time
    B. the concentration of sugar would ultimately become equal in A and B
    C. no diffusion would take place through the membrane
    D. the level in B would become ten times as high as in A
    E. there would be excessive pressure on the membrane

24. Some insects carry disease germs on their bodies and transmit diseases to man merely by contact. Other insects' bodies act as *culture tubes* in which the disease organisms pass a part of their life cycle. 24.___
Which one of these insects is a *culture tube* type of carrier for the disease named after it?

    A. Housefly - tuberculosis   B. Mosquito - malaria
    C. Cockroach - typhoid fever   D. Housefly - common cold
    E. Body louse - typhus fever

25.

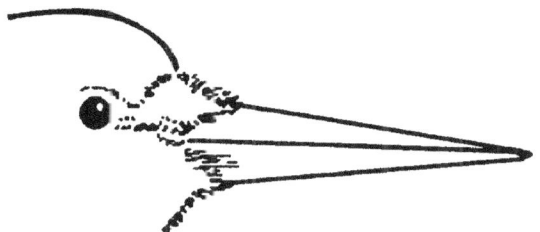

The bird beak shown above is of MOST value to its possessor for

A. crushing seeds
B. drilling for and extracting insects
C. catching fish
D. tearing flesh from bones
E. capturing insects in flight

26. One of the MOST important functions of root hairs is to

A. increase the plant's sensitivity to stimuli
B. enable roots to penetrate deeper into the soil
C. increase the root's total absorbing surface
D. protect the delicate parts of the root from injury
E. increase the total food storage capacity of the root

27. The presence of certain useless structures in man's body, such as the appendix and the muscles in the outer ears, may be an indication that

A. man had a remote ancestor who used these organs
B. man has always been as he is today
C. man can regenerate organs at will
D. these structures have helped man to survive
E. man has undoubtedly descended from the monkey

28. Food is digested in the alimentary tract because

A. the body needs energy
B. food is required for building new cells
C. oxidation would not take place unless the foods were digested
D. man cannot live unless his nutrition requirements are met
E. there are enzymes present which change the food into soluble form

29. Which one of the following traits distinguishes all birds from all reptiles?

A. Birds lay eggs
B. Birds have internal body skeletons
C. Birds are warm-blooded
D. In birds the nerve cord is dorsally located in the body
E. Birds have legs

30. Each secretes hormones EXCEPT the

   A. pituitary gland
   B. lymph nodes
   C. parathyroid glands
   D. adrenal glands
   E. islets of the pancreas

31. Which is an example of sexual reproduction?

   A. Mature yeast plants develop outgrowths which, when shed, are the young yeast plants.
   B. A mature paramecium divides into two offspring.
   C. A fish hatchery worker pours some salmon milt into a jar of salmon eggs which later hatch into young salmon.
   D. A gardener plants pieces of potatoes containing *eyes* and later harvests a crop of potatoes.
   E. A fern plant produces many brown spores on the undersides of the leaves. These spores give rise to young plants.

32. It is sometimes desirable to mix a small amount of white clover seed with the grass seed when seeding a new lawn because the clover

   A. furnishes shade to the young grass plants when they first come up
   B. tends to crowd out weeds
   C. produces carbon dioxide
   D. protects the young grass plants from injury until the sod is well established
   E. has root structures which harbor nitrogen-fixing bacteria

33. A _____ is *cold-blooded*.

   A. frog
   B. goose
   C. bat
   D. whale
   E. polar bear

34. One of the MOST marked differences between animal cells and plant cells is that

   A. plant cells have chromosomes
   B. animal cells ordinarily have a nucleus
   C. animal cells contain protoplasm
   D. animal cells have a variety of shapes
   E. plant cells usually have thick, rigid walls

35. Blood flowing through the pulmonary veins is distinguished from blood flowing through the large jugular vein in the neck region in that the blood in the pulmonary veins

   A. carries disease-resisting substances known as antibodies
   B. contains nutrient substances, such as sugar, fats, and amino acids
   C. has more white blood cells
   D. carries a fresh supply of oxygen
   E. has a higher concentration of carbon dioxide

36. A group of organisms protected by a *suit of armor* is

   A. sponges
   B. arthropods
   C. amphibians
   D. roundworms
   E. primates

37. All EXCEPT _____ constitute real homes for living things.   37._____

    A. the oceans
    B. inland ponds and lakes
    C. the air over the earth
    D. swiftly flowing fresh-water streams
    E. the land mass of the earth

38. Why can a green plant continue to carry on photosynthesis after the oxygen surrounding   38._____
    it has been removed by a chemical absorbing agent?

    A. Green plants do not use oxygen.
    B. Green plants use carbon dioxide in respiration.
    C. Transpiration serves the same function in green plants as respiration does in animals.
    D. Green plants use nitrogen instead of oxygen.
    E. Green plants release free oxygen as a by-product in food manufacturing.

39. Four of the following offer evidence that living things have gone through long ages of   39._____
    gradual development on the earth.
    Which one does NOT offer evidence supporting this theory?

    A. Many fossils of animals and plants show series of changes from simple to complex forms.
    B. The whale has bones, which suggest that its ancestors may have had legs.
    C. A very young human embryo is hardly distinguishable from a very young fish embryo.
    D. The hand and arm of a man are similar, bone for bone, to the forefoot and foreleg of a horse.
    E. There is only one species of mankind living upon the earth at the present time.

40.   40._____

    The above skeleton indicates that the animal belonged to the _____ group.

    A. roundworm   B. arthropod   C. echinoderm
    D. chordate   E. mollusk

41. The GREATEST disturbers of the balance of nature have been   41._____

    A. the carnivorous animals
    B. the insects
    C. civilized people
    D. volcanoes and earthquakes
    E. bacteria and fungi

42. The Mediterranean fruit fly has eight chromosomes in each of its body cells. The normal number of chromosomes in one of its sperm cells or egg cells would, therefore, be

    A. two
    B. four
    C. eight
    D. sixteen
    E. thirty-two

43. A characteristic of the offspring of asexual reproduction is that they

    A. are apt to resemble each other and the parent more closely than is true of the offspring of sexual reproduction
    B. differ markedly from each other in hereditary traits
    C. are likely to show many mutations
    D. can adapt themselves better to changing environmental conditions than the offspring of sexual reproduction
    E. are very unpredictable as to the physical and genetic traits they will possess

44. Bone tissue is hard because

    A. the body needs a strong, rigid supporting framework
    B. the possession of an internal skeleton distinguishes the chordates from all other phyla of animals
    C. the muscles require places for attachment in order to function properly
    D. it is needed to protect delicate parts of the body from injury
    E. calcium compounds are deposited in the spaces between and around the cells

45. *So we may doubt whether, in cheese and timber, worms are generated or if beetles and wasps in cow dung, or if butterflies, shellfish, eels, and such life be procreated of putrefied matter. To question this is to question reason, sense, and experience. If he doubts this, let him go to Egypt, and there he will find the fields swarming with mice begot of the mud of the Nile, to the great calamity of the inhabitants.*
    In the above paragraph, the theory under question is that of

    A. sexual reproduction
    B. special creation
    C. spontaneous generation
    D. vegetative reproduction
    E. regeneration

46. The wings of India's *dead leaf* butterfly are shaped like a leaf and the undersides are colored like a dead leaf. This butterfly is an example of

    A. symbiosis
    B. protective resemblance
    C. warning coloration
    D. metamorphosis
    E. None of these

47. If you are about the right weight, the BEST way for you to stay that way is to

    A. exercise every day
    B. eat meals that contain enough vitamins and minerals
    C. cut out all desserts and snacks
    D. adjust your calorie intake to your calorie needs
    E. None of the above

48. It has been observed that increasing the amount of x-irradiation increases the number of mutations per thousand irradiated organisms.
Which graph indicates this process?

A.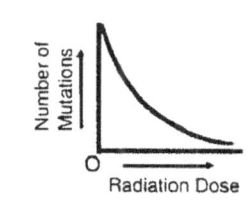

B.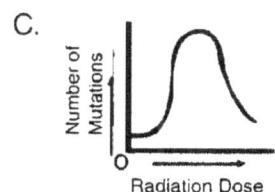

C. (Number of Mutations vs Radiation Dose, bell-shaped curve)

D. (Number of Mutations vs Radiation Dose, horizontal line)

E. None of the above

49. Beans were growing in one garden patch and asparagus was growing in another adjacent patch. Equal amounts of salt were added to the soil in both patches. All of the beans died, and all of the asparagus lived.
Which is the MOST acceptable explanation for these observations?

   A. Asparagus plants can tolerate larger amounts of salt than beans can.
   B. Asparagus plants use the salt to build tissue.
   C. Some substance other than salt killed the beans.
   D. Bean plants do not need as much water as asparagus plants do.
   E. None of the above

50.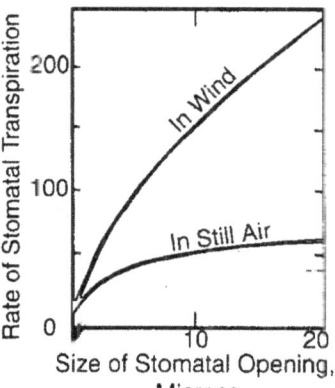

The above graph describes corn plants with equal areas of leaf surface.
A plant in _____ would PROBABLY lose water fastest.

   A. wind, stomatal openings 10 microns
   B. wind, stomatal openings 15 microns
   C. still air, stomatal openings 10 microns
   D. still air, openings 20 microns
   E. None of the above

KEY (CORRECT ANSWERS)

1. B	11. A	21. B	31. C	41. C
2. C	12. A	22. E	32. E	42. B
3. A	13. B	23. B	33. A	43. A
4. A	14. A	24. B	34. E	44. E
5. E	15. C	25. B	35. D	45. C
6. C	16. B	26. C	36. B	46. B
7. D	17. D	27. A	37. C	47. D
8. C	18. C	28. E	38. E	48. A
9. D	19. E	29. C	39. E	49. A
10. E	20. B	30. B	40. D	50. B

TEST 2

DIRECTIONS: Each question or incomplete statement is followed by several suggested answers or completions. Select the one that BEST answers the question or completes the statement. *PRINT THE LETTER OF THE CORRECT ANSWER IN THE SPACE AT THE RIGHT.*

1. Which one of the following statements regarding the endocrine glands is TRUE? 1.____

    A. The removal of any endocrine gland will cause death.
    B. Overactivity of a gland produces effects similar to those produced by underactivity.
    C. Large numbers of different kinds of hormones may be found in the alimentary canal.
    D. Overactivity of a gland may always be corrected by the administration of a synthetic hormone.
    E. The activity of one gland is often affected by the products of others.

2. Differences in genetic composition in similar-appearing individuals may be discovered experimentally by 2.____

    A. the use of x-rays
    B. the use of hormones
    C. a back-cross
    D. crossing-over
    E. regeneration

3. The variety of present day forms of animals and plants may be reasonably explained on the basis that 3.____

    A. each form has been specially created
    B. present forms have resulted from effort on the part of individual organisms to adapt themselves to changing environments
    C. any environmental change always produces structural changes that are hereditary
    D. all new forms are better fitted for survival than their predecessors
    E. all present forms have developed as results of variations that have occurred in previous generations

4. The parathyroid glands in man are important because certain processes in them influence the 4.____

    A. concentration of calcium in the blood
    B. metabolism of carbohydrates
    C. rate of growth
    D. sodium and potassium balance in the blood
    E. oxidative metabolism

5. Enzymes differ from inorganic catalysts in that enzymes 5.____

    A. are more resistant to extremes of temperature
    B. must be present in greater concentration to be effective
    C. are most effective at temperatures of about 212° F
    D. catalyze only specific reactions
    E. cannot be obtained in crystalline form

6. Chemical compounds in dead organisms are transformed into compounds usable by plants CHIEFLY by the action of

   A. inorganic elements in soil
   B. saprophytic bacteria and fungi
   C. parasitic fungi
   D. unicellular animals
   E. pathogenic microorganisms

7. Exchange of material between two homologous chromosomes in synapsis is known as

   A. fertilization
   B. linkage
   C. crossing-over
   D. hybridization
   E. cleavage

8. A person born with an underactive anterior lobe of the pituitary gland is LIKELY to be

   A. a cretin
   B. a giant
   C. a midget
   D. feeble-minded
   E. diabetic

9. The GREATEST amount of heat energy will be furnished to the body by complete oxidation of one gram of

   A. glucose
   B. sucrose
   C. starch
   D. fat
   E. protein

10. Inactivation of the vagus nerve results in

    A. an acceleration of the heart beat
    B. blindness
    C. loss of sensation of pain
    D. an increase in the flow of saliva
    E. impairment of the sense of taste

11. An animal's intelligence is correlated CHIEFLY with

    A. its ability to form conditioned reflexes
    B. the complexity of its pattern of instinctive behavior
    C. the sum of all its simple reflex actions
    D. the usefulness to the animal of its instinctive behavior
    E. the keenness of its sense organs

12. One difference between the nutrition of higher animals and plants is the relatively larger proportion of the animal's food

    A. used in the synthesis of carbohydrates
    B. used in the synthesis of organic components of protoplasm
    C. used in the synthesis of supporting tissue
    D. stored within the organism
    E. oxidized

13. During the development of a fruit from a flower, an ovule becomes the

    A. entire fruit
    B. fleshy part of the fruit
    C. endosperm
    D. embryo
    E. seed

14. The GREATEST degree of precipitation will be obtained when rabbit blood serum which has been immunized against human blood serum is mixed with diluted blood serum of   14._____

    A. non-immunized rabbits   B. squirrels
    C. monkeys   D. man-like apes
    E. man

15. A disease which might be contracted from some food that an individual has eaten is   15._____

    A. typhus fever   B. anemia   C. diabetes
    D. trichinosis   E. ringworm

16. *The evidence seems to show beyond question that our present species of plants have descended...from simpler and fewer species which formerly existed—back, to a single kind which throve in remotest antiquity.*
On the basis of this statement alone, it might follow that   16._____

    A. the number of species of plants is decreasing
    B. generally speaking, plants are becoming simpler
    C. an organism could become so complex that its very complexity would lead to its extinction
    D. the number of species of plants is increasing
    E. ancient plants were more successful than modern plants

17. An example of a flowering plant is a(n)   17._____

    A. fern   B. mushroom   C. moss
    D. arbor vitae   E. corn

18. An individual could continue to live a fairly normal life after the removal or destruction of any EXCEPT one   18._____

    A. adrenal gland   B. kidney
    C. lung   D. cerebral hemisphere
    E. parathyroid gland

19. Two well-watered geranium plants, in sealed pots, were placed under two dry bell jars, X and Y. The leaves of the plant under Jar X were coated with vaseline on both upper and lower surfaces, while those of the plant under Jar Y were not coated. The two bell jars were then placed in bright sunlight for 8 hours.
At the end of this time, what was the condition of the inside surface of the bell jars?   19._____

    A. Jar X showed less moisture than Jar Y.
    B. Jar X showed more moisture than Jar Y.
    C. Each jar was perfectly dry.
    D. Each jar was very moist with no noticeable difference in amount.
    E. Jar X was covered with many fine droplets of vaseline.

20. A man is able to maintain his balance when he sits, stands, or walks PRIMARILY because of the functioning of the   20._____

    A. medulla oblongata connecting the brain and the spinal cord
    B. adrenal glands secreting adrenalin into the blood stream
    C. spinal cord
    D. solar plexus or nerve center in the stomach region of the abdomen
    E. semicircular canals in the ears

21. What is the MOST important reason for cutting many branches off a deciduous tree that is to be transplanted? It

    A. prevents too great a water loss until the roots are reestablished
    B. tends to reduce the rate of photosynthesis
    C. increases the rate of water absorption
    D. increases the efficiency of food production
    E. exposes more surface to the atmosphere

22. When a sip of water goes *down the wrong way*, there is improper functioning of the

    A. larynx   B. trachea   C. pharynx
    D. epiglottis   E. Eustachian tubes

23. Wheat is planted three years in succession in Field X, while soybeans are planted three years in succession in Field Y.
    The soil nitrogen will PROBABLY

    A. increase in Field X
    B. increase in Field Y
    C. decrease in Field Y
    D. decrease equally in both fields
    E. be unaffected in either field

Questions 24-26.

DIRECTIONS: For each of Questions 24 through 26, select the organism that belongs to a different phylum from the other four.

24. A. Sunfish   B. Starfish   C. Trout
    D. Bass   E. Codfish

25. A. Pine   B. Sunflower   C. Oak
    D. Fern   E. Dandelion

26. A. Ameba   B. Paramecium   C. Euglena
    D. Malarial parasite E. Hydra

27. On the basis of photosynthesis and conditions necessary for this process to occur, it should be possible to produce a marked increase in plant growth in a closed greenhouse room by

    A. slowly releasing a continuous supply of carbon dioxide into the room from a carbon dioxide tank
    B. drying the air in the room with a calcium chloride apparatus
    C. providing electric light during the day in addition to the usual sunlight
    D. uncapping a bottle containing a chlorophyll solution and allowing its vapors to pass into the air in the room
    E. slowly releasing a continuous supply of pure oxygen into the room from an oxygen tank

28. External fertilization in animals is MOST often associated with

   A. a land habitat
   B. small size
   C. parental care of the young
   D. asexual reproduction
   E. living in water

29. Which statement might BEST account for the fact that the trout, which is a very active fish, is most frequently found in the swift, well-churned type of stream?

   A. Swiftly flowing water contains less decaying organic matter.
   B. The trout escapes most of its natural enemies by living in the rapids.
   C. Water in the rapids is more highly oxygenated than relatively still water.
   D. Food is more easily caught in a swiftly flowing stream.
   E. The trout gets considerable satisfaction from skirting danger.

30. When blood passes through the pancreas, the amount of _____ in the blood _____.

   A. digestive enzyme; increases
   B. insulin; increases
   C. sugar; increases
   D. adrenalin; increases
   E. hormone; decreases

31. The scientific name of the leopard frog is *Rana pipiens* and that of the bullfrog is *Rana catesbiana*.
    These scientific names indicate that both frogs belong to the same

   A. genus   B. species   C. class   D. order   E. family

32. Wheat rust can be eliminated BEST by

   A. dusting wheat fields with insect poisons
   B. encouraging ladybird beetles to multiply rapidly
   C. spreading lime on the fields before plowing
   D. getting rid of all common barberry bushes in the vicinity
   E. draining the swamps and wet lands in that region

Questions 33-39.

DIRECTIONS: Questions 33 through 39 are on the MOST effective measures for preventing certain diseases. For each disease named, select from the following KEY the best preventive.

33. Yellow fever

KEY
A. Water treatment and milk pasteurization
B. Eradication of insect carriers
C. An addition to or a subtraction from one's diet
D. Immunization, such as vaccination or inoculation
E. Eugenics

34. Anemia

35. Diphtheria

36. Rabies

37. Rickets

38. Night blindness

39. Undulant fever

Questions 40-43.

DIRECTIONS: For Questions 40 through 43, select from the following KEY the scientific classification which might be applied to each statement.

KEY
A. Generalization
B. Problem
C. Fact by definition
D. Hypothesis
E. Fact by demonstration

40. Would an orchardist who raises cherries for the market consider the robin a harmful or a beneficial bird? 40.___

41. The robin may have developed in antiquity from reptile ancestors. 41.___

42. Why do robins migrate to southern latitudes in the winter? 42.___

43. All members of the thrush family of birds have spotted breasts, either in the young or in the adult stage. 43.___

44. According to current theories, what is the order in which the following plants appeared on Earth, the earliest listed FIRST? 44.___
    I. Ferns
    II. Angiosperms
    III. Algae
    The CORRECT answer is:

    A. I, II, III   B. I, III, II   C. II, I, III
    D. III, I, II   E. II, III, I

45. In a kidney transplant, a person would have the BEST chance for the organ to be accepted by his body if the kidney came from his 45.___

    A. brother   B. fraternal twin   C. mother
    D. identical twin   E. father

46.

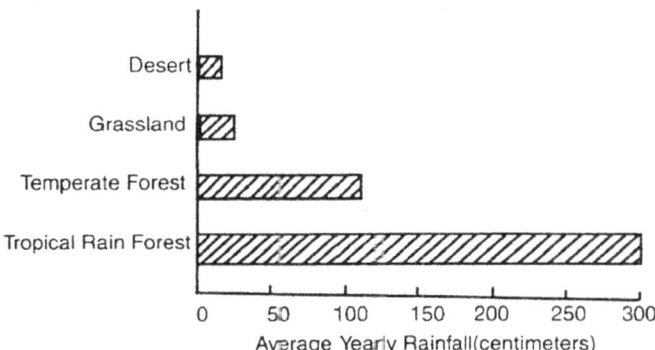

Identify the conclusion MOST closely related to the information presented in the above graph.

A. There is a relationship between temperature and the types of plants existing in an ecosystem.
B. The amount of available water is a factor that determines the types of plants growing in a region.
C. Areas of limited rainfall have the widest variety of plants.
D. There is a relationship between latitude and the types of plants existing in an ecosystem.
E. None of the above

Questions 47-48.

DIRECTIONS: Questions 47 and 48 are to be answered on the basis of the following graph.

BODY TEMPERATURE OF FOUR SPECIES OF ANIMALS
AT VARIOUS EXTERNAL TEMPERATURE

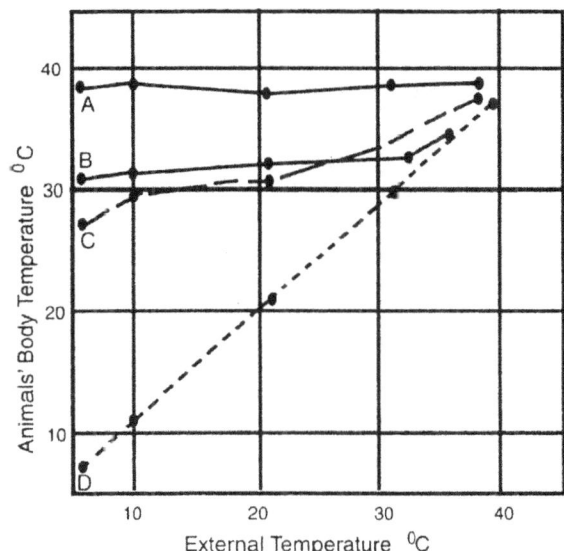

47. Which curve represents a cold-blooded animal?

A. A
B. B
C. C
D. D
E. None of these

48. Which curve represents an animal that is warm-blooded and whose temperature is LEAST affected by changes in external temperature?

    A. A   B. B   C. C
    D. D   E. None of the above

48.____

Questions 49-50.

DIRECTIONS: Questions 49 and 50 are to be answered on the basis of the following illustration.

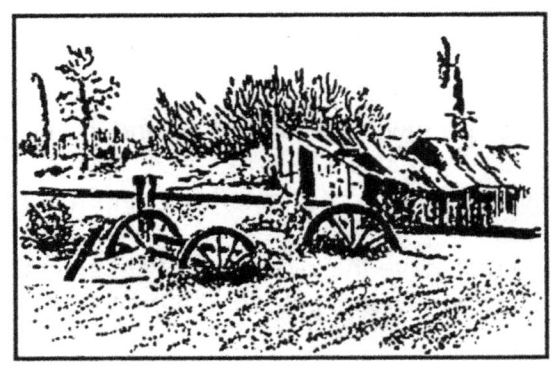

49. In the scene above, _____ has occurred.

    A. a dust storm   B. sheet erosion
    C. gullying   D. a snowstorm
    E. a flood

49.____

50. The MOST probable cause of this occurrence was

    A. overgrazing range land followed by floods
    B. forest removal followed by heavy rains
    C. a sudden drop in temperature followed by high winds
    D. a forest fire
    E. wheat farming on dry plains followed by high winds

50.____

KEY (CORRECT ANSWERS)

1. E	11. A	21. A	31. A	41. D
2. C	12. E	22. D	32. D	42. B
3. E	13. E	23. B	33. B	43. A
4. A	14. E	24. B	34. C	44. D
5. D	15. D	25. D	35. D	45. D
6. B	16. D	26. E	36. D	46. B
7. C	17. E	27. A	37. C	47. D
8. C	18. D	28. E	38. C	48. A
9. D	19. A	29. C	39. A	49. A
10. A	20. E	30. B	40. B	50. E

TEST 3

DIRECTIONS: Each question or incomplete statement is followed by several suggested answers or completions. Select the one that BEST answers the question or completes the statement. *PRINT THE LETTER OF THE CORRECT ANSWER IN THE SPACE AT THE RIGHT.*

1. Three groups of tadpoles of the same age were placed in a bowl containing pond water. The pituitary glands of the tadpoles in Group I were removed; the thyroid glands of the tadpoles in Group II were removed; and the tadpoles of Group II were left intact. In two weeks, only the tadpoles of Group III began to change into frogs.
   These observations are evidence that in frogs, the

   A. thyroid gland controls metamorphosis
   B. pituitary gland controls metamorphosis
   C. pituitary gland controls the thyroid gland
   D. thyroid and pituitary glands are both necessary for metamorphosis
   E. none of the above

2. John said that bean seeds sprout faster in the dark than in the light.
   Of the following, the BEST way for him to test this idea would be to moisten the seeds and then place

   A. some of the seeds in a dark refrigerator and the rest in sunlight
   B. all of the seeds in the sunlight for short periods of time and then move them into the dark
   C. some of the seeds in the dark and the rest in the light at the same temperature
   D. some of the seeds in the ground and the rest under a sunlamp
   E. none of the above

3. Which of the following would account for a fossil oyster found in your backyard?

   A. The oyster was probably fossilized by a volcanic eruption.
   B. Your backyard was probably once under water for a long time.
   C. The earth in your backyard is acid.
   D. The oyster evolved from a water animal to a land form.
   E. None of the above

4. As two students watched two squirrels in a park, the students made specific comments. Which of these comments was an assumption rather than an observation?

   A. The squirrels are getting ready to fight.
   B. One of the squirrels is moving faster than the other.
   C. The squirrels are not the same color.
   D. One of the squirrels dropped his nut.
   E. None of the above

5. The usual biological classification of plants and animals is based PRIMARILY on

   A. age
   B. structure
   C. geographical distribution
   D. size
   E. color

6. The CHIEF reason it is harder to breathe at high altitudes than at low ones is that at high altitudes

   A. the temperatures are lower
   B. there are fewer plants
   C. there is more CO_2
   D. the air pressure is lower
   E. None of the above

7. An animal is surely a bird if it

   A. flies
   B. lays eggs that hatch
   C. has feathers
   D. is warm-blooded
   E. has webbed feet

8. The featherlike gills of most species of fish PRIMARILY provide a

   A. large amount of surface area for the exchange of gases
   B. pump for the rapid flow of blood through the gill filaments
   C. filter for obtaining small particles of food from the water
   D. means for breaking down water into hydrogen and oxygen
   E. None of the above

Questions 9-26.

DIRECTIONS: In each of the following groups of items, there are several statements, phrases, or terms, each of which characterizes or suggests one of the five words or phrases listed above the questions. For each question, select that word or phrase from the above list to which it applies, or with which it is MOST significantly associated, and put the letter of your choice in the space at the right.

Questions 9-11.

   A. Conjugation
   B. Hybridization
   C. Maturation
   D. Inbreeding
   E. Dominance

9. The breeding of parents CLOSELY related to each other.

10. Crossbreeding of parents differing in one or more hereditary characteristics.

11. The appearance of ONLY one of two contrasting characters when the potentialities of both are present in an individual.

Questions 12-14.

    A. Ovum
    B. Uterus
    C. Vagina
    D. Ovary
    E. Oviduct

12. An egg; the female reproductive cell which, after fertilization, develops into a new member of the same species.   12.___

13. An organ in which the eggs or young of animals are retained during embryonic development.   13.___

14. An organ in which animal egg cells are produced.   14.___

Questions 15-17.

    A. Dihybrid
    B. Genotype
    C. Mutant
    D. Phenotype
    E. Homozygote

15. An individual described or recognized by its visible characters WITHOUT reference to its hereditary factors.   15.___

16. An individual whose parents differ with respect to two pairs of hereditary characters.   16.___

17. An individual possessing an abrupt and heritable variation differing from any of its ancestors.   17.___

Questions 18-20.

    A. Taxonomy
    B. Paleontology
    C. Cytology
    D. Anatomy
    E. Ecology

18. The scientific study of organisms of past geological periods, based on fossil remains.   18.___

19. The study of the structures and physiology of cells.   19.___

20. The study of the relations of organisms to each other and to their environment.   20.___

Questions 21-23.

    A. Diastole
    B. Peristalsis
    C. Flexion
    D. Tonus
    E. Extension

21. A wave-like series of muscular contractions, progressing along the walls of various tubes of the body, propelling their contents.

22. A movement that bends one part upon another.

23. The stage of dilation of the heart or relaxation of the heart muscle.

Questions 24-26.

    A. Blood
    B. Neurilemma
    C. Biceps
    D. Neuron
    E. Retina of the eye

24. Epithelial tissue

25. Vascular tissue

26. Muscular tissue

27. Identify the TRUE statement regarding the preservation of animal and plant remains.

    A. The most perfect fossils have been found in metamorphosed rock.
    B. Petrifaction preserves the organism without chemical change.
    C. Most ancient plants and animals ultimately were fossilized.
    D. Complete bodies of large animals have been preserved for thousands of years by low temperatures.
    E. Proterozoic rock is an abundant source of fossils.

28. Injection of pure water into the blood of an animal may indirectly cause its death by

    A. chemical reaction with hemoglobin
    B. plasmolysis of the corpuscles
    C. increasing external pressure upon the corpuscles
    D. swelling and bursting of the corpuscles
    E. destroying the permeability of the plasma membrane of the corpuscles

29. It is probable that the earliest organisms on the earth were MOST similar to present day

    A. saprophytic bacteria or fungi
    B. parasitic bacteria
    C. autophytic (autotrophic) bacteria or simple algae
    D. amoeba-like protozoans
    E. lichens

30. Mitotic cell division takes place

    A. principally in germ cells
    B. more commonly than any other form of cell division in organisms other than the lowest forms
    C. mainly in one-celled organisms
    D. mainly in vertebrates
    E. only under the influence of unfavorable conditions

31. The division of the Class Insecta into orders is made CHIEFLY on the basis of

   A. geographical distribution
   B. complexity of structures
   C. wing structure and mouth parts
   D. size and color
   E. egg-laying habits

32. The diploid number of chromosomes would be found in cells taken from what part of a moss plant?

   A. Archegonium   B. Antheridium   C. Protonema
   D. Calyptra   E. Capsule

33. The existence of cellulose-digesting protozoa in the intestines of termites is an example of

   A. a symbiotic relationship
   B. pathogenic parasitism
   C. saprophytism
   D. ecological succession
   E. a predatory relationship

34. Evidence of man's possible existence in the Pliocene Period is the discovery in sedimentary strata of that period of

   A. crude stone implements or eoliths
   B. crude metallic ornaments
   C. pottery
   D. complete skeletons of man-like creatures
   E. fossil remains of domesticated animals

35. Which one of the following is thought to have borne the GREATEST physical resemblance to man of today?

   A. Pithecanthropus erectus   B. Cro-Magnon man
   C. Neanderthal man   D. Piltdown man
   E. Peking man

36. The evolution of land plants from the Thallophytes to the Spermatophytes has been GENERALLY characterized by a(n)

   A. *decrease* in structural size of the sexual generation
   B. *increase* in the structural size and importance of the sexual generation
   C. *decrease* in the functional importance of the sexual generation
   D. *decreased* dependence on other plants and animals
   E. *decrease* in number of complex structures

37. Colorblindness in man is a recessive sex-linked character. How many of the children of a colorblind mother and a father with normal vision will be colorblind?

   A. All of the children
   B. One-half of the girls and one-half of the boys
   C. All of the girls and none of the boys
   D. All of the boys and none of the girls
   E. None of the children

38. Asphyxiation or suffocation victims are sometimes given a mixture of oxygen and carbon dioxide rather than pure oxygen because the carbon dioxide

   A. stimulates the respiratory center in the medulla
   B. decreases the danger to the victim of a shock resulting from sudden administration of pure oxygen
   C. increases the speed with which gases pass through the lung tissue
   D. decreases the viscosity of the blood
   E. directly stimulates the rib muscles

39. The organism which is LEAST dependent upon other organisms for the procurement of essential food substances is

   A. an amoeba
   B. an autophytic (autotrophic) bacterium
   C. a mushroom
   D. bread mold
   E. man

40. Iodide is added to salt to keep people from developing goiters. The reason for using the iodide is MOST similar to the reason for

   A. applying antiseptic to a cut
   B. taking aspirin for a fever
   C. adding chlorine to water to kill bacteria
   D. adding fluoride to drinking water to prevent tooth decay

41. Which of the following is PROBABLY a drawing of plant cells?

   A.
   B.
   C.
   D.
   E. None of the above

42. The significance of meiosis for heredity lies in which statement?

   A. The great variety of gene combinations that it makes possible
   B. The doubling of the chromosome number in the sex cells of the offspring
   C. The production of offspring identical with the parents
   D. The potential for many offspring
   E. None of the above

43. An experimenter wants to know whether a mouse is more likely to turn left or right in a maze.
Which experimental design is BEST for this purpose?

A.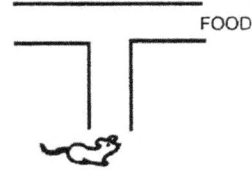

B.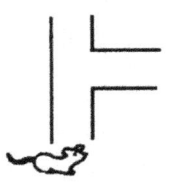

C.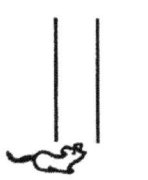

D.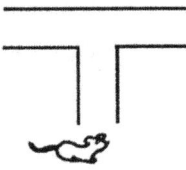

E. None of the above

44. Two plants with pink flowers were crossed, and the following results were obtained: 27 red, 31 white, and 63 pink-flowered plants.
These data indicate that the color of the pink flowers is due to

A. sex-linked recessiveness
B. sex-linked dominance
C. incomplete dominance
D. translocation
E. chromotropsin

45. What is the BEST reason why only consumer organisms and very few producer organisms are found at great ocean depths?

A. In deep water, consumer organisms ingest any producer organisms at a rate that prevents reproduction of the producers.
B. Photosynthesis requires the presence of light.
C. Increased pressure favors the survival of heterotrophs and not of autotrophs.
D. Autotrophs are independent of heterotrophs in deep water.
E. The enormous pressure inhibits growth.

Questions 46-47.

DIRECTIONS: Questions 46 and 47 are to be answered on the basis of the following diagram of the food web.

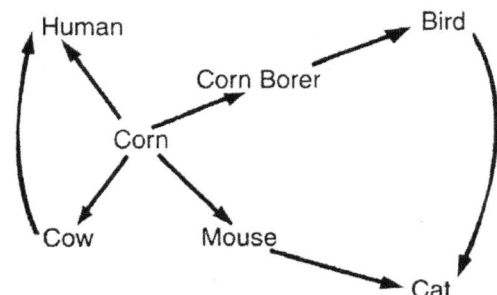

46. Which of these is a PRIMARY producer in this food web?　46._____

　　A. Bird　　B. Cat　　C. Corn　　D. Human　　E. Mouse

47. The food web above includes _____ primary (first-order) consumers?　47._____

　　A. One　　B. Two　　C. Three　　D. Four　　E. Five

Questions 48-50.

DIRECTIONS: Questions 48 through 50 are to be answered on the basis of the following table.

POPULATION RECORDS FOR 9 SPECIES OF BIRDS THAT APPEARED TO BE MOST SERIOUSLY AFFECTED BY APPLICATION OF DDT DUST ON A 40-ACRE PLOT

SPECIES	NO. OF BIRDS COUNTED BEFORE DUSTING	NUMBER OF BIRDS COUNTED DURING FIRST 6 DAYS AFTER DUSTING					
		1st Day	2nd Day	3rd Day	4th Day	5th Day	6th Day
Texas wren	3	2	2	1	0	0	0
Carolina wren	5	1	0	0	0	0	0
Kentucky warbler	1	0	0	0	0	0	0
Yellow-breasted chat	3	0	0	0	0	0	0
Cardinal	10	8	6	5	2	1	1
Blue grosbeak	2	0	0	0	0	0	0
Painted bunting	4	4	3	2	2	0	0
Lark sparrow	8	2	2	2	2	1	1
Field sparrow	5	4	4	4	3	3	1
Total	41	21	17	14	9	5	3

Study the above table and read each question carefully. Then, in the space at the right, mark the letter of your answer according to the KEY below.

KEY
　A. The table tends to support the statement.
　B. The table tends to contradict the statement.
　C. The table furnishes no conclusive evidence, either supporting or contradicting the statement.

48. Within two days after application of DDT to the 40-acre plot, a decrease in numbers was noted in all nine species of birds listed.　48._____

49. Ground-nesting birds were MOST seriously affected by the spreading of DDT over the plot.　49._____

50. DDT MUST be used with extreme caution in areas occupied by birds.　50._____

KEY (CORRECT ANSWERS)

1. D	11. E	21. B	31. C	41. D
2. C	12. A	22. C	32. E	42. A
3. B	13. B	23. A	33. A	43. D
4. A	14. D	24. E	34. A	44. C
5. B	15. D	25. A	35. B	45. B
6. D	16. A	26. C	36. A	46. C
7. C	17. C	27. D	37. D	47. D
8. A	18. B	28. D	38. A	48. A
9. D	19. C	29. C	39. B	49. C
10. B	20. E	30. B	40. D	50. A

EXAMINATION SECTION
TEST 1

DIRECTIONS: Each question or incomplete statement is followed by several suggested answers or completions. Select the one that BEST answers the question or completes the statement. *PRINT THE LETTER OF THE CORRECT ANSWER IN THE SPACE AT THE RIGHT.*

1. Blood type O can be transfused to anyone because it contains

    A. serum A antibodies *only*
    B. serum B antigens *only*
    C. neither antigens nor antibodies
    D. both antigens and antibodies

2. Point mutations are those involving

    A. a large segment of a chromosome
    B. a small number of DNA base pairs
    C. deletions of chromosome segments
    D. insertions of many DNA molecules

3. Enzymes are BEST described as

    A. cell division inhibitors
    B. cell division activators
    C. inorganic catalysts
    D. organic catalysts

4. The development of an egg WITHOUT fertilization is known as

    A. meiosis   B. oogenesis
    C. parthenogenesis   D. gametogenesis

5. Intracellular digestion is the function of the

    A. contractile vacuole   B. episome
    C. centrosome   D. lysosome

6. The maintenance of the same genotype in successive generations of a species is associated with

    A. internal fertilization   B. external fertilization
    C. sexual reproduction   D. asexual reproduction

7. Metamorphosis is demonstrated by the reproductive patterns of the

    A. hydra and amoeba
    B. alligator and axolotyl
    C. frog and blowfly
    D. grasshopper and earthworm

8. The operon is a(n)

    A. group of structural genes that code for enzymes
    B. group of chromosomes that carry homologous genes

C. activated strip of mRNA
D. inducer molecule that increases the production of enzymes

9. Sperm and eggs of the same species are *identical* in

   A. size and number
   B. shape and motility
   C. chromosome number
   D. amount of cytoplasm

10. One muscle pulls a bone in one direction and another muscle pulls it back. This is known as

    A. synergistic activity
    B. antagonistic activity
    C. active transport
    D. passive transport

11. When reproduction occurs by budding,

    A. there is unequal division of chromosomes
    B. the parent cell remains
    C. daughter cells replace the parent cell
    D. there is no DNA replication

12. Muscle is connected to bone by means of

    A. ligaments
    B. myofibrils
    C. muscle fibers
    D. tendons

13. During the light reactions of photosynthesis,

    A. water molecules are split
    B. carbon dioxide molecules are split
    C. carbon dioxide combines with hydrogen
    D. carbon combines with water

14. Mitochondria are organelles which

    A. are necessary for the process of diffusion to take place
    B. are found in the nucleus of some cells
    C. initiate cell division in living cells
    D. contain respiratory enzymes

15. Diffusion is a process in which

    A. molecules move from a region of high concentration to one of low concentration
    B. molecules move from a region of low concentration to one of high concentration
    C. the same number of molecules move in opposite directions
    D. molecules move randomly

16. In lichens, algae and fungi form a relationship known as

    A. parasitism
    B. saprophytism
    C. predation
    D. mutualism

17. The white-eyed condition in fruit flies results from

    A. sex linkage
    B. crossing over
    C. mutation
    D. dominent genes

18. Of the following steps in mitosis, the event occurring first is

    A. replication of chromosomes
    B. disappearance of the nuclear membrane
    C. separation or the centrosomes
    D. appearance of the spindle

19. DNA molecules that are NOT attached to bacterial chromosomes are known as

    A. plastids
    B. plasmids
    C. desmids
    D. plasmodesmata

20. The contractile units of muscle fibers are

    A. flame cells
    B. myofibrils
    C. nerve endings
    D. sinews

21. Eutrophication of a lake

    A. may be accelerated by increased phosphorus input
    B. is caused by the addition of copper sulfate to reduce algae blooms
    C. increases the salinity of the lake
    D. can be prevented by laws governing thermal pollution

22. The molarity of a solution that contains 2 g NaOH per 100 ml of solution is (Na=23, O=16, H=1)

    A. 0.05
    B. 0.20
    C. 0.50
    D. 1.00

23. Of the following, the equation which represents a double replacement reaction is

    A. $Ca + Cl_2 \rightarrow CaCl_2$
    B. $2Na + 2H_2O \rightarrow H_2 + 2NaOH$
    C. $2HgO \rightarrow 2Hg + O_2$
    D. $BaCl_2 + Na_2SO_4 \rightarrow BaSO_4 + 2NaCl$

24. The colligative property MOST useful in determining molecular weights of large molecules is

    A. boiling point elevation
    B. freezing point depression
    C. vapor pressure lowering
    D. osmotic pressure

25. A solution which maintains an *almost constant* pH on addition of acid or base is said to be

    A. inert
    B. buffered
    C. neutral
    D. stable

26. In the reaction of $CuS + H_2 \rightarrow Cu + H_2S$, the substance oxidized is

    A. CuS
    B. H_2
    C. Cu
    D. H_2S

27. Of the following, the SAFEST student preparation of oxygen is

   A. electrolysis of water
   B. catalytic decomposition of household hydrogen peroxide
   C. heating $KClO_3$ with MnO_2
   D. adding water to sodium peroxide

28. The TOTAL number of atoms in a molecule of $(NH_4)_4Fe(CN)_6 \cdot 3H_2O$ is

   A. 16   B. 22   C. 24   D. 42

29. When the equation $Al + Fe_3O_4 \rightarrow Al_2O_3 + Fe$ is properly balanced, the coefficient of Fe_3O_4 is

   A. 1   B. 2   C. 3   D. 4

30. Carbon-14 dating may be used to

   A. determine the age of a specimen
   B. measure the life span of a carbon atom
   C. determine how long it takes for carbon to return to the atmosphere
   D. measure the half-life of carbon

KEY (CORRECT ANSWERS)

1. C	11. C	21. A
2. B	12. D	22. A
3. D	13. A	23. D
4. C	14. D	24. B
5. D	15. A	25. B
6. D	16. D	26. B
7. C	17. A	27. B
8. A	18. A	28. D
9. C	19. A	29. C
10. B	20. B	30. A

TEST 2

DIRECTIONS: Each question or incomplete statement is followed by several suggested answers or completions. Select the one that BEST answers the question or completes the statement. *PRINT THE LETTER OF THE CORRECT ANSWER IN THE SPACE AT THE RIGHT.*

1. A solution pf pH 8.5 is considered to be

   A. weakly acidic
   B. strongly acidic
   C. weakly basic
   D. strongly basic

2. All known samples of a given substance contain 70% Fe and 30% O. The substance is *probably* a(n)

   A. compound
   B. mixture
   C. element
   D. solid solution

3. The number of grams in a pound is *approximately*

   A. 2.2   B. 30   C. 450   D. 2200

4. The formula for ferric oxide is

   A. Fe_2O B. FeO_2 C. FeC D. Fe_2O_3

5. An element has the following numbers of electrons in its electron shells: 2-8-8-2. The BEST description of this element is that it

   A. forms an ion with a charge of +2
   B. is a non-metal
   C. can accept two electrons
   D. forms a negative ion

6. A 1 molal solution of NaCl has a LOWER freezing point than a 1 molal solution of glucose ($C_6H_{12}O_6$) because

   A. each mole of NaCl forms two moles of particles in solution
   B. NaCl has greater chemical activity
   C. NaCl decomposes on freezing
   D. glucose contains hydrogen and oxygen in the same proportions as water

7. $^{16}_{8}O$ and $^{18}_{8}O$ are known as

   A. isobars
   B. isomers
   C. isomorphs
   D. isotopes

8. Each of the following are allotropes EXCEPT

   A. oxygen- ozone
   B. monoclinic and rhombic sulfur
   C. red and white phosphorus
   D. iron II and iron III

9. The molecular formula for a saturated hydrocarbon compound (alkane) is
   A. CH
   B. C_nH_{2n}
   C. C_nH_{2n+2}
   D. C_nH_{2n-2}

10. To be liquefied by compression, CO_2 must be at or below its critical
    A. temperature
    B. size
    C. mass
    D. density

11. A suitable source of current for a classroom demonstration of the Hoffman apparatus may be obtained from the 110 volt AC line and a
    A. transformer *only*
    B. transformer and rectifer
    C. rectifier *only*
    D. transformer and resistor

12. Addition of 10 g of NaOH to a liter of water will cause the GREATEST change in
    A. density
    B. boiling point
    C. viscosity
    D. pH

13. The oxidation number of chlorine in the compound $KClO_4$ is
    A. +7
    B. +3
    C. -1
    D. +1

14. A nanogram is
    A. 10^{-6}g
    B. 10^{-9}g
    C. 10^{-12}g
    D. 10^{-15}g

15. The properties of a permanent magnet are *currently* explained by the theory of
    A. domains
    B. permeability
    C. hysteresis
    D. electron mobility

16. The resistance of a 60 watt lamp designed to operate in a 120 volt circuit is _____ ohms.
    A. 0.5
    B. 2
    C. 120
    D. 240

17. The ferromagnetic elements are
    A. iron, copper and nickel
    B. aluminum, iron and cobalt
    C. iron, cobalt and nickel
    D. aluminum, iron and copper

18. As resistors are added in parallel to circuit, the TOTAL resistance of the circuit
    A. increases
    B. decreases, then increases
    C. decreases
    D. remains the same

19. Two blocks of metal are placed in contact. Heat will flow from one to the other ONLY if they
    A. have different specific heats
    B. are of different materials

C. contain different amounts of internal energy
D. are at different temperatures

20. The IDEAL mechanical advantage of a pulley system can be determined by

    A. counting the number of strands of rope supporting the resistance
    B. calculating the ratio of resistance to effort
    C. calculating the ratio of effort to resistance
    D. counting the number of pulleys in the system

21. When carbon rods connected to a battery are immersed in a copper sulfate solution, a reddish brown coating forms on

    A. both the positive and negative electrode
    B. the positive electrode
    C. neither electrode
    D. the negative electrode

22. The transfer of heat by motion of hot material is called

    A. conduction B. convection
    C. radiation   D. advection

23. In calibrating a thermometer, it is necessary to mark

    A. the freezing point *only*
    B. the boiling point *only*
    C. both the freezing and boiling points
    D. both the freezing and melting points

24. The image formed by a lens is a point image when the object is at

    A. infinity
    B. a distance between one and two focal lengths
    C. a distance twice the focal length
    D. a distance equal to the focal length

25. A 12 volt source is connected to a circuit containing resistances of 2 ohms and 4 ohms in series. The current in the circuit is _____ amperes.

    A. 6   B. 2   C. 3   D. 8

26. Two lamps are identical except that the filament in lamp A is thicker than in lamp In identical circuits, _____ will be brighter because it has _____ resistance.

    A. A, more   B. B, more
    C. A, less   D. B, less

27. When two positively charged pith balls are brought close together, they _____ each other.

    A. repel
    B. have no effect on
    C. attract
    D. first repel and then attract

28. As the speed of a magnet moving in a coil of wire *increases*, the current induced in the coil 28.___

    A. *decreases* then *increases*
    B. *decreases*
    C. *increases*
    D. remains the same

29. If sound travels at 330 meters per second, the wavelength, in meters, of a sound wave of frequency 1000 hertz is 29.___

    A. 0.33   B. 33   C. 3.0   D. 330,000

30. If the frequency of a sound wave *increases*, there is an *increase* the 30.___

    A. length of the sound wave
    B. pitch of the sound
    C. loudness of the sound
    D. velocity of the sound wave

KEY (CORRECT ANSWERS)

1. C	11. B	21. D
2. A	12. D	22. B
3. C	13. A	23. C
4. D	14. B	24. A
5. A	15. A	25. B
6. A	16. D	26. B
7. D	17. C	27. A
8. D	18. C	28. C
9. C	19. D	29. C
10. C	20. A	30. B

TEST 3

DIRECTIONS: Each question or incomplete statement is followed by several suggested answers or completions. Select the one that BEST answers the question or completes the statement. *PRINT THE LETTER OF THE CORRECT ANSWER IN THE SPACE AT THE RIGHT.*

1. The usefulness of laser light is due to its

   A. monochromaticity
   B. coherence
   C. collimation
   D. high frequency

2. A magnet can be produced by

   A. stroking a magnetic material in one direction with a magnet
   B. stroking a magnetic material in both directions with a magnet
   C. freezing a magnetic material
   D. heating a magnetic material

3. A cube of wood has a density of 0.6 grams per cubic centimeter. When placed in alcohol (specific gravity 0.8), what percentage of the block will be submerged?

   A. 25   B. 67   C. 75   D. 80

4. The transverse nature of light waves is BEST demonstrated by the phenomenon of

   A. refraction
   B. polarization
   C. interference
   D. reflection

5. A temperature of 40° Celsius is equal to a temperature on the Fahrenheit scale of

   A. 75°   B. 100°   C. 104°   D. 120°

6. A 4-meter pole is used to lift a 100 kilogram crat When the fulcrum is one meter from the crate end of the pole, the IDEAL mechanical advantage is

   A. 1   B. 2   C. 3   D. 4

7. When a body is immersed in a fluid, the fluid exerts an upward force

   A. equal to the weight of the displaced fluid
   B. greater than the weight of the displaced fluid
   C. less than the weight of the displaced fluid
   D. equal to the weight of the body in air

8. An example of a chemically formed rock is

   A. granite
   B. sandstone
   C. gypsum
   D. shale

9. Karst topography is *most closely* associated with

   A. earthquakes
   B. glacial development
   C. wave actions
   D. ground water

10. An instrument used to determine relative humidity is the

A. hygrometer	B. hydrometer
C. barometer	D. anemometer

11. The Foucault experiment demonstrates the

    A. earth's rotation on its axis
    B. relative motion of the planets
    C. earth's revolution around the sun
    D. moon's revolution around the earth

12. The outer atmosphere of the sun is the

A. chromosphere	B. photosphere
C. troposphere	D. corona

13. The MOST important biological result of the weathering of rock is the

A. formation of soil	B. release of oxygen
C. production of gravel	D. leaching which occurs

14. The cloud type that *immediately* precedes the passage of a cold front is

A. stratus	B. altostratus
C. nimbostratus	D. cumulonimbus

15. The type of precipitation associated with air currents is

A. sleet	B. snow
C. drizzle	D. hail

16. Earthquakes originate at the

A. focus	B. epicenter
C. Moho	D. core

17. To determine longitude, it is necessary to know both local time and

    A. the altitude of polaris
    B. the time of day at the Prime Meridian
    C. your elevation above sea level
    D. the radius of the earth at apparent noon

18. The factors MOST responsible for the erosive action of a stream are its volume of water and

    A. the length of its channel
    B. its slope
    C. the direction of its flow
    D. the temperature of the water

19. The half-life of a given substance is 1000 years. After 2000 years, 10 grams of this substance would have decayed to _____ grams.

    A. 0   B. 0.5   C. 2.5   D. 5

20. The two igneous rocks that are the MAJOR components of both continental and oceanic crusts are

A. granite and basalt B. gneiss and marble
C. slate and sandstone D. schist and gabbro

21. Evidence that the continents have drifted apart may be found in

    A. ocean mineral deposits
    B. magnetic patterns in rocks
    C. molten materials in young moutains
    D. sea caves along the coast

22. The *primary* source of energy for ocean currents, winds and waves is

    A. movement of the earth's crust
    B. solar radiation reaching the earth
    C. rotation of the earth
    D. movement in the troposphere

23. The *probable* source area for a mTw air mass is

    A. North Pacific B. Canada
    C. Gulf of Mexico D. Hudson Bay

24. The type of rock *most closely* associated with fossils is

    A. igneous
    B. banded metamorphic
    C. distorted banded metamorphic
    D. sedimentary

25. Potential energy is stored as latent heat when

    A. water evaporates from lakes
    B. rain falls from clouds
    C. clouds form from radiational cooling
    D. fog forms from radiational cooling

26. As molten material cools, the size of the crystals in the igneous rock formed depends upon the

    A. amount of iron present
    B. amount of silica present
    C. rate at which gases are dissolved in the material
    D. rate at which the material cools

27. Barchans are features associated with the erosional force of

    A. winds B. waves
    C. glaciers D. rivers

28. Given equal geographic areas, which of the following would absorb the MOST solar radiation on a summer day?

    A. Lake B. Glacier
    C. Forest D. Sandy Beach

29. A cloud may form when moist air rises because

A. the air pressure increases
B. the dew point increases
C. additional water vapor is added to the air
D. the air is cooled to or below its dewpoint

30. Winds in the northern hemisphere are cyclonic due to 30.____

A. high pressure
B. Coriolis effect
C. air masses
D. weather fronts within the cyclone

KEY (CORRECT ANSWERS)

1. B	11. A	21. B
2. A	12. D	22. B
3. C	13. A	23. C
4. B	14. D	24. D
5. C	15. D	25. A
6. C	16. B	26. D
7. A	17. B	27. A
8. C	18. B	28. C
9. D	19. C	29. D
10. A	20. A	30. B

EXAMINATION SECTION
TEST 1

DIRECTIONS: Each question or incomplete statement is followed by several suggested answers or completions. Select the one that BEST answers the question or completes the statement. *PRINT THE LETTER OF THE CORRECT ANSWER IN THE SPACE AT THE RIGHT.*

1. Pressure builds up in a tire on a hot day because 1.____

   A. the tire expands
   B. air is added
   C. the gaseous molecules have more energy at higher temperatures
   D. a chemical reaction takes place
   E. oxygen sublimes

2. $-218°$ C can be expressed as 2.____

   A. $218°$ K   B. $55°$K   C. $491°$ K   D. $273°$ K   E. $-218°$ F

3. Of the following substances the one with the HIGHEST heat of vaporization is 3.____

   A. helium   B. hydrogen   C. oxygen
   D. hydrogen sulfide   E. water

4. A solution of a salt gives a yellow flame test and forms a white precipitate when treated with $AgNO_3$. 4.____
   The solution contained

   A. KBr   B. NaI   C. NaCl   D. NaBr   E. KCl

5. An element that forms ionic solids with hydrogen is 5.____

   A. nitrogen   B. oxygen   C. carbon
   D. arsenic   E. sodium

6. Freshly boiled water tastes flat. 6.____
   This is due to the

   A. presence of salts in the water
   B. removal of salts from the water
   C. removal of dissolved gases from the water
   D. destruction of organisms present in the water
   E. increased solubility of carbon dioxide in water at the elevated temperatures

7. Of the following list of metals, the one MOST abundant in the earth's crust is 7.____

   A. iron   B. lead   C. tin
   D. copper   E. aluminum

8. A sample of hydrogen is collected over water at a temperature of $20°$ C. The vapor pressure of water is 17.5 mm of Hg at this temperature. The pressure of the sample is equalized against atmospheric pressure which is 750 mm of Hg. 8.____
   The pressure of the hydrogen in the tube is _____ mm Hg.

   A. 730   B. 732.5   C. 760   D. 767.5   E. 770

9. Solid sodium chloride will NOT conduct an electric current due to the fact that

   A. sodium chloride is a covalent compound
   B. the sodium and chloride ions are not free to move in the solid
   C. chlorine is very electronegative
   D. sodium chloride is insoluble
   E. sodium chloride contains ions

10. The empirical formula of a substance is CH_2. Five and six tenth grams of the substance has a volume of 2.24 liters at standard temperature and pressure. The molecular formula is

    A. CH_2 B. C_2H_4 C. C_3H_6 D. C_4H_8 E. C_5H_{10}

11. Two liters of 2.0 molar K_2CrO_4 contains

    A. 1 mole K_2CrO_4
    B. 2 moles K_2CrO_4
    C. 4.0 moles K_2CrO_4
    D. 194 grams K_2CrO_4
    E. 388 grams K_2CrO_4

12. The molecular weight of H_2SO_4 is (atomic weights H, 1; S, 32; O, 16)

    A. 49 B. 50 C. 97 D. 98 E. 196

13. Carbon (atomic weight 12) reacts with oxygen to form carbon dioxide. What weight of carbon reacts with 4 grams of oxygen? _____ gram(s)

    A. 1 B. 1.5 C. 3 D. 4 E. 12

14. An element identified in the sun's atmosphere before it was found on earth was

    A. hydrogen   B. helium   C. silicon
    D. magnesium   E. titanium

15. When a liquid evaporates, one observes a cooling effect. This is accounted for by

    A. the liquid being wet
    B. energy being required to convert a liquid to a gas
    C. movement of air
    D. the conversion of liquid to gas being an exothermic process
    E. energy being liberated when a liquid is converted to a gas

16. Given $H_{2(g)} + Br_{2(l)} = 2HBr_{(g)} + 17.2$ kilocalories, the heat liberated when .5 mole hydrogen reacts with .5 mole bromine is _____ kilocalories.

    A. .5 B. 1 C. 8.6 D. 17.2 E. 34.4

17. If the combustion of 1 gram of methane raises the temperature of 2 liters of water 6.65° C., the heat of combustion of the methane is

    A. 6.65 calories/gram methane
    B. 13.3 calories/gram methane
    C. 6.65 kilocalories/gram methane
    D. 13.3 kilocalories/gram methane
    E. 6.65 kilocalories/mole methane

18. There is danger of explosion of dry, powdered combustible matter due to   18._____

   A. the large surface area of the material
   B. the absence of moisture
   C. the combustible nature of the substance
   D. static electricity
   E. the high concentration of the powdered substance

19. For two gases in a container at room temperature, their rate of reaction will be increased   19._____
    by

   A. increasing the temperature
   B. addition of a catalyst
   C. addition of one of the gases
   D. increasing the pressure
   E. all the preceding procedures

20. It is difficult to *hard boil* an egg at high elevations due to   20._____

   A. water boiling at a lower temperature when pressure is reduced
   B. less oxygen in the air at high elevations
   C. the water boils too vigorously
   D. water boils at a higher temperature at higher elevations
   E. the humidity is too low

Questions 21-25

DIRECTIONS: An assumed atom has the following structure: the nucleus contains 13 protons and 14 neutrons

21. The atomic weight is   21._____

   A. 13   B. 14   C. 26   D. 27   E. 28

22. The atomic number is   22._____

   A. 13   B. 14   C. 26   D. 27   E. 28

23. A common oxidation number of the element is   23._____

   A. +1   B. +2   C. +3   D. +4   E. +5

24. The predicted compound of the above element which we shall represent as A with oxygen would be   24._____

   A. A_2O B. AO C. A_2O_3 D. AO_2 E. A_2O_5

25. The symbolism $_{11}Na^{23}$ indicates that the nucleus of this isotope of sodium contains   25._____

   A. 11 protons and 23 neutrons
   B. 11 protons and 12 neutrons
   C. 12 protons and 11 neutrons
   D. 23 protons and 23 neutrons
   E. 23 electrons

KEY (CORRECT ANSWERS)

1.	C	11.	C
2.	B	12.	D
3.	E	13.	B
4.	C	14.	B
5.	E	15.	B
6.	C	16.	C
7.	E	17.	D
8.	B	18.	A
9.	B	19.	E
10.	D	20.	A

21. D
22. A
23. C
24. C
25. B

TEST 2

DIRECTIONS: Each question or incomplete statement is followed by several suggested answers or completions. Select the one that *BEST* answers the question or completes the statement. *PRINT THE LETTER OF THE CORRECT ANSWER IN THE SPACE AT THE RIGHT.*

1. A substance that exists *mainly* as molecules when dissolved in water is

    A. table salt
    B. sulfuric acid
    C. sodium hydroxide
    D. sugar
    E. sodium peroxide

2. The solubility product for Ag_2S is equal to

    A. $2(Ag+2) + (S^=)$
    B. $(Ag^+) + (S^=)$
    C. $(Ag^+)(S^=)$
    D. $(Ag^+)_2(S^=)$
    E. $2(Ag^+)^2(S^=)$

3. An example of a weak acid is _____ acid.

    A. hydrochloric
    B. nitric
    C. acetic
    D. sulfuric
    E. perchloric

4. Hydrogen sulfide (a weak acid of formula H_2S) reacts with water to form mainly

    A. $H_3O^+ + S^=$
    B. $H^+ + S^=$
    C. $HsO^+ + HS^-$
    D. $H^+ + HS^-$
    E. $H_3S+ + OH^-$

5. In pure water at 25° C, the concentration of hydronium ion (hydrogen ion) is _____ moles(s)/liter.

    A. 10^{-14} B. 10^{-7} C. 10^{-5} D. 1   E. 7

6. A container suitable for storage of aqueous solutions of $CuSO_4$ could be made of

    A. zinc
    B. iron
    C. copper
    D. mercury
    E. lead

7. With what volume of .600 normal NaOH would 100 ml of .150 normal sulfuric acid react? _____ ml.

    A. 25.0   B. 50.0   C. 100   D. 200   E. 400

8. The numerical value of the vapor pressure of water at its boiling point is _____ mm of Hg.

    A. 22.4   B. 100   C. 224   D. 760   E. 1000

9. If tens grams of ice at 0° C is converted to liquid water at 0° C, it requires _____ calories.

    A. 10   B. 80   C. 540   D. 800   E. 5400

10. A salt solution is boiling. As the water boils away, the temperature

    A. is 100 degrees centigrade
    B. remains constant
    C. decreases
    D. increases
    E. depends on the source of heat

11. Two clear liquids, when mixed with each other, yield a solid and a liquid. This represents

    A. neutralization
    B. precipitation
    C. purification
    D. sublimation
    E. homogenization

12. A solution would be classified as strongly acid if it exhibited a pH of

    A. 0   B. 4   C. 7   D. 10   E. 14

13. A one tenth normal solution of H_2SO_4 would exhibit a pH of

    A. 1   B. 4   C. 7   D. 10   E. 13

14. A one tenth normal solution of sodium chloride would exhibit a pH of

    A. 1   B. 4   C. 7   D. 10   E. 13

15. A one tenth normal solution of ammonia would exhibit a pH of *approximately*

    A. 1   B. 3   C. 7   D. 11   E. 13

16. In the electrolysis of a concentrated sodium chloride solution, the substance produced at the positive electrode is

    A. sodium
    B. sodium hydroxide
    C. chlorine
    D. hydrogen
    E. sodium chloride

17. Silver chloride will dissolve in ammonia solution because

    A. ammonia is a base
    B. the silver ammonia complex ion is formed
    C. of the common ion effect
    D. chlorine is an active nonmetal
    E. double decomposition reaction can occur

18. Acetone, CH_3COCH_3, would be classified as a(n)

    A. hydrocarbon
    B. ether
    C. ester
    D. aldehyde
    E. ketone

19. A vegetable oil would be classified as a(n)

    A. hydrocarbon
    B. ether
    C. ester
    D. aldehyde
    E. ketone

20. A lubricating oil would be classified as a(n)

    A. hydrocarbon
    B. ether
    C. ester
    D. aldehyde
    E. ketone

21. The following compound, CH₃OH, would be classified as a(n) 21._____

    A. hydrocarbon   B. ether   C. ester
    D. aldehyde   E. phenol

22. The class of compound to which CH₃COOH belongs is? 22._____

    A. acid   B. alcohol   C. phenol
    D. ester   E. amide

23. _____ produces the GREATEST lowering of the freezing point when a molecular or formula weight of the substance is dissolved in 1000 grams of water. 23._____

    A. C₁₂H₂₂O₁₁   B. C₂H₅OH   C. CaCl₂
    D. NaCl   E. HCl

24. A metal that is noted for its low density and good electrical conductivity is 24._____

    A. Fe   B. Cu   C. Al   D. Ag   E. Ni

25. In the preparation of chlorine by reaction of hydrochloric acid with manganese dioxide, the number that appears in front of HCl in the balanced equation is 25._____

    A. 1   B. 2   C. 3   D. 4   E. none of the above

KEY (CORRECT ANSWERS)

1. D
2. D
3. C
4. C
5. B

6. C
7. A
8. D
9. D
10. D

11. B
12. A
13. A
14. C
15. D

16. C
17. B
18. E
19. C
20. A

21. D
22. A
23. C
24. C
25. D

TEST 3

DIRECTIONS: Each question or incomplete statement is followed by several suggested answers or completions. Select the one that BEST answers the question or completes the statement. PRINT THE LETTER OF THE CORRECT ANSWER IN THE SPACE AT THE RIGHT.

1. The formula $CuSO_4 \cdot 5H_2O$ represents a compound containing   1.___

   A. carbon B. uranium C. sodium
   D. sulfur E. none of these

2. Potassium sulfate would be classified as a(n)   2.___

   A. element B. nonpolar compound C. mixture
   D. acid E. salt

3. An element in the same family of the periodic table as potassium that would be predicted to be more active than potassium is   3.___

   A. Li B. Rb C. Bi
   D. F E. none of these

4. The predicted formula for the compound of sodium and sulfur is   4.___

   A. Na_2S B. Na_S C. NaS_2 D. Na_2S_3 E. NaS_6

5. The predicted formula for the compound of nitrogen and hydrogen would be   5.___

   A. HN B. H_2N C. NH_3 D. NH_4 E. NH_5

6. The predicted formula for the compound of phosphorus and oxygen would be   6.___

   A. P_2O B. PO C. PO_2 D. P_2O_4 E. P_2O_5

7. Hydrogen is *often* prepared by reacting zinc with   7.___

   A. CH_4 B. H_2O C. H_3O^+ D. H_2O_2 E. NH_3

8. The MOST active nonmetal is   8.___

   A. oxygen B. fluorine C. chlorine
   D. iodine E. sulfur

9. A water solution of which of the following materials would turn pink litmus blue?   9.___

   A. NH_3 B. C_2H_5OH C. HCl D. CH_3COOH E. SO_3

10. The reaction of a nonmetallic oxide with water produces a(n)   10.___

    A. salt B. base C. acid
    D. anhydride E. alcohol

11. The MOST abundant element is   11.___

    A. silicon B. iron C. aluminum
    D. oxygen E. hydrogen

12. When SO_2 dissolves in water the product is   12._____

    A. sulfuric acid   B. sulfurous acid
    C. hydrosulfuric acid   D. hyposulfurous acid
    E. sulfite

13. Air is composed of 80%   13._____

    A. oxygen   B. nitrogen   C. carbon dioxide
    D. water vapor on a humid day   E. hydrogen

14. Which of the following will react with bromine?   14._____

    A. NaCl   B. KI   C. CCl_4 D. He   E. NaBr

15. Frash devised a method of mining   15._____

    A. salt   B. sulfur   C. iron
    D. oil   E. coal

16. The chemical properties of the elements are a periodic function of their   16._____

    A. atomic weight   B. molecular weight
    C. atomic number   D. melting point
    E. boiling point

17. The calcium salt of $HClO_3$ would be named calcium _____.   17._____

    A. chloride   B. hypochlorite   C. chlorite
    D. chlorate   E. perchlorate

18. The acid found in soft drinks is   18._____

    A. HCl   B. H_2SO_4 C. H_2C_O3
    D. C_2H_5OH E. H_2S

19. One liter is about the same as one   19._____

    A. pint   B. quart   C. gallon
    D. cubic centimeter   E. cubic foot

20. Which is largest?   20._____

    A. Millimeter   B. Liter   C. Kiloliter
    D. Centiliter   E. Microliter

21. In a mixture of salt and water, salt is the   21._____

    A. solute   B. solvent   C. solution
    D. coloid   E. acid

22. When hydrogen burns it forms   22._____

    A. water   B. carbon dioxide
    C. carbon monoxide   D. hydrogen peroxide
    E. all of these

23. Commercial oxygen is prepared from

    A. H_2O B. liquid air   C. $KCLO_3$
    D. Fe_2O_3 E. $NaClO_4$

24. In the reaction of ethane, C_2H_6, with oxygen, the number that appears in front of O_2 in the balanced equation is

    A. 1   B. 2   C. 3
    D. 4   E. none of the above

25. Concentrated sulfuric acid can be transported in iron containers because

    A. iron is below hydrogen in the activity series
    B. concentrated sulfuric acid contains very little hydronium ion
    C. iron forms a protective oxide coat
    D. sulfuric acid is very dense
    E. sulfuric acid is a dehydrating agent

KEY (CORRECT ANSWERS)

1. D
2. E
3. B
4. A
5. C

6. E
7. C
8. B
9. A
10. C

11. D
12. B
13. B
14. B
15. B

16. C
17. D
18. C
19. B
20. C

21. A
22. A
23. B
24. E
25. B

TEST 4

DIRECTIONS: Each question or incomplete statement is followed by several suggested answers or completions. Select the one that *BEST* answers the question or completes the statement. *PRINT THE LETTER OF THE CORRECT ANSWER IN THE SPACE AT THE RIGHT.*

1. Which electron arrangement represents that of an active metal? 1.____
    A. 2   B. 2 8   C. 2 8 1   D. 2 8 4   E. 2 8 7

2. Oxygen may be prepared by 2.____
    A. heating a carbonate
    B. reacting an acid with an active metal
    C. heating potassium chloride
    D. electrolysis of water
    E. reacting a metallic oxide with water

3. A crystal of solid solute is added to a solution. More crystals form. The solution was 3.____
    A. unsaturated   B. saturated   C. supersaturated
    D. dilute   E. normal

4. Manganese dioxide is *often* used in small amounts in the laboratory preparation of oxygen because 4.____
    A. it is a cheap source of oxygen
    B. it serves as a catalyst for the decomposition of potassium chlorate
    C. historically, it is the compound from which oxygen was prepared
    D. it is a commercial source of oxygen
    E. all metal oxides are good sources of oxygen

5. Calcium oxide would react as a(n) 5.____
    A. acid   B. acid anhydride   C. base
    D. active metal   E. proton donor

6. The oxidation number of chlorine in $KClO_3$ is 6.____
    A. -1   B. +4   C. +5   D. +7   E. +1

7. The valence of calcium in $Ca_3(PO_4)_2$ is 7.____
    A. +1   B. +2   C. +3   D. +4   E. +6

8. Dilute sulfuric acid reacts with barium chloride because 8.____
    A. it is an acid
    B. it contains hydronium ion
    C. an ionic product can be formed
    D. incoluble $BaSO_4$ can be formed
    E. this is a method for preparation of hydrochloric acid

9. The molecular weight of $Fe_2(SO_4)_3$ is

   A. 152　　B. 208　　C. 272　　D. 336　　E. 400

10. The formula of sodium sulfate is

    A. $SoSO_3$　　B. $NaSO_4$　　C. Na_2SO_4　　D. $NaSO_3$　　E. NaS

11. Strontium, which is in the same family as calcium, would be predicted to exhibit a valence of

    A. +1　　B. +2　　C. +3　　D. +4　　E. +5

12. Which one of the following elements would be *most likely* to be found as components of compounds in nature?

    A. Argon　　　　　　　　B. Copper　　　　　　　　C. Gold
    D. Sodium　　　　　　　 E. All of these occur naturally as compounds

13. An electron arrangement that represents an inert element is

    A. 282　　B. 24　　C. 287　　D. 288　　E. 283

14. The electron arrangement *most likely* to represent an amphoteric element is

    A. 281　　B. 282　　C. 283　　D. 287　　E. 288

15. The symbol for potassium is

    A. P　　B. Po　　C. K　　D. Ka　　E. Pa

16. The class of compound to which H_2SO_4 belongs is

    A. acid　　　　　　　　B. base　　　　　　　　C. sulfide
    D. salt　　　　　　　　 E. anhydride

17. In solid sodium chloride, the bond between sodium and chlorine is best classified as a(n) _____ bond.

    A. ionic　　　　　　　　B. covalent　　　　　　　C. coordinate covalent
    D. metallic　　　　　　 E. hydrogen

18. In gaseous hydrogen chloride, the bond between hydrogen and chlorine is best classified as a(n) _____ bond.

    A. hydrogen　　　　　　B. covalent　　　　　　　C. coordinate covalent
    D. metallic　　　　　　 E. ionic

19. A property that is characteristic of a low molecular weight covalent compound is

    A. high boiling point
    B. good electrolyte
    C. high heat of vaporization
    D. usually solid at room temperature
    E. none of these

20. A vegetable oil may be changed to a solid by

    A. raising the temperature
    B. reacting with hydrogen
    C. hydrolysis
    D. treatment with an antioxidant
    E. by all of these methods

21. An element in the same family of the periodic table as chlorine and that is *more* active than chlorine is

    A. iodine   B. sodium   C. oxygen
    D. fluorine   E. carbon

22. A water would be classified as hard if it contained

    A. sodium ion   B. chloride ion
    C. magnesium ion   D. potassium ion
    E. iron

23. Hydrogen, deuterium, and tritium are

    A. isotopes   B. allotropes
    C. isomers   D. resonance hybrids
    E. chemically unrelated

24. There is danger of explosion of dry, powdered, combustible matter due to the

    A. large surface area of the material
    B. absence of moisture
    C. combustible nature of the substance
    D. static electricity
    E. high concentration of the powdered substance

25. In the neutralization of phosphoric acid with sodium hydroxide, the number that appears in front of NaOH in the balanced equation is

    A. 1   B. 2
    C. 3   D. 4
    E. none of the above

KEY (CORRECT ANSWERS)

1.	C	11.	B
2.	D	12.	D
3.	C	13.	D
4.	B	14.	C
5.	C	15.	C
6.	C	16.	A
7.	B	17.	A
8.	D	18.	B
9.	E	19.	E
10.	C	20.	B

21. D
22. C
23. A
24. A
25. C

EXAMINATION SECTION
TEST 1

DIRECTIONS: Each question or incomplete statement is followed by several suggested answers or completions. Select the one that BEST answers the question or completes the statement. PRINT THE LETTER OF THE CORRECT ANSWER IN THE SPACE AT THE RIGHT.

1. Iron pyrites are iron

    A. oxides
    B. sulfides
    C. carbonates
    D. sulfates
    E. chlorides

2. The gas which has the odor of rotten eggs is

    A. CH_4
    B. H_2
    C. H_2S
    D. SO_2
    E. CS_2

3. A paint turns black in the presence of sulfides if it contains

    A. lead carbonate
    B. zinc oxide
    C. titanium oxide
    D. cadmium carbonate
    E. arsenous oxide

4. Bauxite is the ore of

    A. mercury
    B. magnesium
    C. lead
    D. copper
    E. aluminum

5. The process of heating heavier hydrocarbon molecules under pressure to split them is

    A. polymerization
    B. hydrogenation
    C. reduction
    D. cracking
    E. sublimation

6. All organic molecules contain the element

    A. sulfur
    B. carbon
    C. oxygen
    D. chlorine
    E. nitrogen

7. The Haber process is used in the manufacture of

    A. sodium carbonate
    B. ammonia
    C. nitric acid
    D. sulfuric acid
    E. sulfur

8. Common table sugar is

    A. glucose
    B. fructose
    C. sucrose
    D. galactose
    E. lactose

9. Amino acids are the building blocks of

    A. starch
    B. cellulose
    C. sugar
    D. fat
    E. protein

10. Concentrated nitric acid is used to test for

    A. starch
    B. cellulose
    C. sugar
    D. fat
    E. protein

11. A permanent type of antifreeze suitable for car radiators is

   A. sodium chloride
   B. carbon tetrachloride
   C. ethyl alcohol
   D. ethylene glycol
   E. acetic acid

12. Cryolite is used in refining

   A. iron
   B. copper
   C. G. aluminum
   D. tin
   E. chromium

13. A break-up of a nucleus into two almost equal parts is

   A. half-life
   B. fusion
   C. fission
   D. chain reaction
   E. transmutation

14. The MOST penetrating radiation of radioactive elements is

   A. alpha particles
   B. beta particles
   C. gamma rays
   D. neutrons
   E. ultra violet rays

15. When a base and a fat react, a product formed is

   A. water
   B. hydrogen
   C. soap
   D. acid
   E. oxygen

16. The number of electrons in the first energy level of an atom never exceeds

   A. 1   B. 2   C. 6   D. 8   E. 16

17. An example of a basic salt is

   A. $NaHSO_4$
   B. $AlCl_3$
   C. K_2SO_4
   D. $NaAL(SO_4)_2$
   E. $Pb_2(OH)_2CO_3$

18. The compound predicted to exist as a liquid at the HIGHEST temperature is

   A. C_4H_{10}
   B. CH_3OCH_3
   C. CH_3CHO
   D. $CH_3CH_2CH_2OH$
   E. CH_4

19. The compound predicted to give water solutions of acidic pH is

   A. NaCL   B. NH_3 C. Na_2CO_3 D. KOH   E. $AlCl_3$

20. The compound predicted to give water solutions of most acidic pH is

   A. CH_3COOH
   B. CH_3CH_2OH
   C. CH_3CONH_2
   D. $CH_2ClCOOH$
   E. CCl_3COOH

21. The formula $C_{17}H_{35}COONa$ represents a compound containing

   A. nitrogen
   B. three different elements
   C. four different elements

D. five different elements
E. six different elements

22. A compound composed of 40 percent calcium and 12 percent carbon could have the formula 22.____

   A. CaC   B. CaC_2 C. $CaCO_2$ D. $CaCO_3$ E. CaC_2O_4

23. Hydrogen may be prepared by reacting an acid with 23.____

   A. copper   B. sodium hydroxide   C. water
   D. zinc   E. aluminum oxide

24. Which of these elements would be *most likely* to be found in the free state? 24.____

   A. Al   B. Zn   C. Mg   D. K   E. Ag

25. The water solution ____ would turn pink litmus blue. 25.____

   A. HCL   B. SO_2 C. CO_2 D. NH_3 E. SO_3

KEY (CORRECT ANSWERS)

1. B
2. C
3. A
4. E
5. D

6. B
7. B
8. C
9. E
10. E

11. D
12. C
13. C
14. C
15. C

16. B
17. E
18. D
19. E
20. E

21. C
22. D
23. D
24. E
25. D

TEST 2

DIRECTIONS: Each question or incomplete statement is followed by several suggested answers or completions. Select the one that BEST answers the question or completes the statement. PRINT THE LETTER OF THE CORRECT ANSWER IN THE SPACE AT THE RIGHT.

1. The oxidation number of oxygen in K_2O is

    A. 2   B. 1   C. 0   D. -1   E. -2

2. The oxidation number of sulfur in $Na_2S_2O_3$ is

    A. -2   B. 0   C. 2   D. 4   E. 6

3. A mathematical expression for the equilibrium constant for the following reaction $2NH_{3(g)} = N_{2(g)} + 3H_{2(g)}$ is

    A. $\dfrac{(N_2)(H_2)^3}{(NH_3)^2}$

    B. $\dfrac{(NH_3)^2}{(N_2)(H_2)^3}$

    C. $\dfrac{2(NH_3)}{(N_2)+3(H_2)}$

    D. $\dfrac{(N_2)+3(H_2)}{2(NH_3)}$

    E. $\dfrac{(N_2)(H_2)}{(NH_3)}$

4. The ratio of air to hydrogen which would react MOST completely is

    A. one to one
    B. one part air to two parts hydrogen
    C. two parts air to one part hydrogen
    D. two 1/2 parts air to one part hydrogen
    E. ten parts air to one part hydrogen

5. The formula of the salt formed when iron reacts with sulfuric acid is

    A. $FeSO_4$ B. FeS C. $FeSO_3$
    D. $Fe_2(SO_4)_3$ E. $Fe_2(SO_3)_3$

6. For the reaction $2NH_{3(g)} = N_{2(g)} + 3H_{2(g)}$ an INCREASE in pressure would

    A. decrease the reaction rates
    B. cause some NH_3 to decompose to establish equilibrium
    C. decrease the yield of N_2 and H_2 at equilibrium
    D. have no effect on equilibrium concentrations of reactants and products
    E. catalyze the reaction

7. The weight of HCl (molecular weight 36.5) that is present in 2.0 liters of 6.0 molar solution is _____ grams.

   A. 2.0　　　　　　B. 6.0　　　　　　C. 12.0
   D. 36.5　　　　　 E. none of these

8. A metal that will NOT react with acids to form hydrogen gas and a salt is

   A. Zn　　B. Fe　　C. Al　　D. Na　　E. Cu

9. A metal that will react with cold water to form hydrogen gas and a base is

   A. Zn　　B. Fe　　C. Al　　D. Na　　E. Cu

10. The molecular weight of $Na_2SO_4 \cdot 10H_2O$ is

    A. 87　　　　　B. 176　　　　C. 274
    D. 322　　　　 E. none of the above

11. An example of a pure substance is

    A. river water　　　　　　　B. milk
    C. potassium perchlorate　　D. all of these
    E. none of these

12. In *general*, metals

    A. have low melting points
    B. have negative oxidation numbers
    C. will all displace hydrogen from dilute acid solutions
    D. are nonconductors
    E. transfer electrons readily

13. Oxygen is prepared commercially from

    A. H_gO　　　　B. BaO_2　　　　C. liquid air
    D. Na_2O_2　　 E. $KClO_3$

14. Sugar is decomposed by sulfuric acid because sulfuric acid is a(n)

    A. oxidizing acid　　　B. dehydrating agent
    C. dense liquid　　　　D. strong acid
    E. nonvolatile liquid

15. A water solution of which of the following substances is classified as an acid?

    A. SO_2　　B. CH_4　　C. NH_3　　D. CaO　　E. Na_2O_2

16. An oxidizing agent

    A. *always* contains oxygen
    B. is *always* reduced in a redox reaction
    C. *always* donates electrons
    D. is a catalyst
    E. is *always* a metal

17. For the following reaction at equilibrium $2SO_{2(g)} + O_{2(g)} = 2SO_{3(g)}$ + heat, the yield of SO$_3$ would Be increased by

    A. *increasing* the temperature
    B. *ncreasing* the pressure
    C. *deareasing* the concentration of SO$_2$
    D. *adding* a catalyst
    E. *decreasing* the concentration of O$_2$

18. An element forming an ion resembling the electronic structure of $_2He^4$ is

    A. $_1H^1$
    B. $_8O^{16}$
    C. $_{11}Na^{23}$
    D. $_{17}Cl^{35}$
    E. $_{10}Ne^{20}$

19. The oxidation number of sulfur is +4 in which ONE of the following compounds?

    A. H$_2$S
    B. SO$_2$
    C. Na$_2$S$_2$O$_3$
    D. H$_2$SO$_4$
    E. CS$_2$

20. Isotopes differ by the

    A. number of electrons in the K energy level
    B. charge on the nucleus
    C. mass of the nucleus
    D. oxidation number
    E. number of electrons in the outermost energy level

21. A Lewis acid is

    A. ALWAYS a proton donor
    B. an elebtron pair acceptor
    C. an electron pair donor
    D. a substance that always yields aqueous hydrogen ions
    E. one classification of bromide ion

22. An example of a polar compound is

    A. CH$_4$
    B. H$_2$O
    C. CCl$_4$
    D. CO$_2$
    E. CS$_2$

23. A precipitate will be observed for a dilute aqueous solution containing

    A. Na$^+$ Cl$^-$, NO$_3^-$, K$^+$
    B. NH$_4^+$, NO$_3^-$, Br$^-$, Mg^{++}
    C. Ca^{++}, Cl$^-$, NO$_3^-$, Ba^{++}
    D. Ag$^+$, Cl$^-$, NO$_3^-$, Na$^+$
    E. Na$^+$, SO$_4^=$, H$^+$, Cl$^-$

24. A substance that contains a coordinate covalent bond is

    A. H$_2$O
    B. NaCl
    C. NH$_3$
    D. H$_2$SO$_4$
    E. O$_2$

25. An example of an oxidation reduction reaction is

    A. $SO_2 + H_2O = H_2SO_3$
    B. $BaCl_2 + H_2SO_4 = BaSO_4 + 2HCl$
    C. $2FeCl_2 + Cl_2 = FeCl_3$
    D. $H_2SO_4 + ZnO = ZnSO_4 + H_2O$
    E. $2H_2O = H_3O^+ + OH^-$

25.____

KEY CORRECT ANSWER

1.	E	11.	C
2.	C	12.	E
3.	A	13.	C
4.	D	14.	B
5.	A	15.	A
6.	C	16.	B
7.	E	17.	B
8.	E	18.	A
9.	D	19.	B
10.	D	20.	C
21.	B		
22.	B		
23.	D		
24.	D		
25.	C		

TEST 3

DIRECTIONS: Each question or incomplete statement is followed by several suggested answers or completions. Select the one that *BEST* answers the question or completes the statement. *PRINT THE LETTER OF THE CORRECT ANSWER IN THE SPACE AT THE RIGHT.*

1. One would predict that zinc would react with dilute sulfuric acid as

    A. zinc sulfate is a salt
    B. water would be formed
    C. zinc is above hydrogen in the activity series
    D. sulfuric acid is a strong oxidizing agent
    E. zinc sulfate is water soluble

2. When sodium reacts with water

    A. the hydrogen ion concentration of the solution is increased
    B. oxygen is evolved
    C. hydrogen is evolved
    D. neutralization occurs
    E. hydrogen peroxide is formed

3. When sodium carbonate reacts with hydrochloric acid

    A. carbon dioxide is evolved
    B. hydrogen is evolved
    C. oxygen is evolved
    D. sodium chloride precipitates
    E. moist pink litmus would be turned blue by the gas evolved

4. An example of a polar compound is

    A. O_2 B. HCl   C. CCl_4 D. C_2H_6 E. CO_2

5. The compound that would be predicted to exhibit the HIGHEST solubility in water is

    A. O_2 B. CH_4 C. CH_3OH
    D. CCl_4 E. C_4H_9OH

6. Of the following, the change that would slow the rate of a chemical reaction is

    A. addition of a catalyst
    B. a decrease in temperature
    C. an increase of pressure if the reaction is between gases
    D. an increase in concentration of one reactant
    E. all of the above

7. An element that forms an ion with the same electron configuration as $2He^4$ is

    A. $_1H^1$ B. $_8O^{16}$ C. $_{11}Na^{23}$
    D. $_{17}Cl^{35}$ E. $_{10}Ne^{20}$

8. The SMALLEST particle of a compound that retains the properties of the compound is a(n)

    A. molecule
    B. ion
    C. gram molecular weight
    D. atom
    E. gram atomic weight

9. The PRINCIPAL reason for using a pressure cooker in cooking is to increase the rate of chemical reaction by

    A. *increasing the* temperature of the contents
    B. *increasing* -the pressure of the gaseous reactants
    C. *increasing* the surface area of the reactants *protecting* the contents from air
    D. *adding* a catalyst

10. Which of the following conditions describes an atom of aluminum ($_{13}Al^{27}$)?

    A. 3 valence electrons
    B. 13 neutrons and 14 protons in nucleus
    C. electron arrangement 2 8 1 3 2
    D. electron arrangement 2 8 8 8 1
    E. 5 valence electrons

11. Which of the following conditions describes an atom of bromine ($_{35}Br^{80}$)? _____ in nucleus

    A. 35 neutrons and 45 protons
    B. 35 neutrons and 45 electrons
    C. 45 neutrons and 35 protons
    D. 80 neutrons
    E. 80 protons

12. When entering into chemical combination, the majority of atoms with two electrons in their outermost orbit will ____ electron(s).

    A. gain two
    B. gain six
    C. share eight
    D. lose one
    E. lose two

13. The positively charged particle in an atom is

    A. proton
    B. electron
    C. beta particle
    D. neutron
    E. gamma ray

14. Fish can live in water because they

    A. do not need oxygen
    B. can use the oxygen that is united with the hydrogen in H_2O.
    C. use oxygen dissolved in water
    D. use CO_2 dissolved in water
    E. can float on water

15. In the reaction of HCl with MnO_2 to produce chlorine, the chlorine in HCl is

    A. oxidized
    B. reduced
    C. neutralized
    D. hydrolized
    E. ionized

16. When NaOH reacts with ferric sulfate, one of the products of the reaction is

    A. $Fe(OH)_3$ B. $Fe(OH)_2$ C. H_2O D. SO_2 E. H_2

17. In the reaction of $Al(OH)_3$ and H_2SO_4, one of the products is

    A. H_2 B. Al   C. S   D. H_2O E. O_2

18. For the reaction $NaClO_4$ → $NaCl + O_2$ the coefficient that would appear in front of oxygen in the balanced equation is

    A. 1   B. 2   C. 3   D. 4   E. 5

19. For the reaction $Ca(OH)_2 + CO_2 \rightarrow CaCO_3 + H_2O$, the coefficient that would appear in front of H_2O in the balanced equation is

    A. 1   B. 2   C. 3   D. 4   E. 5

20. For the reaction $Al_2O_3 + HCl \rightarrow AlCl_3 + H_2O$, the coefficient that would appear in front of H_2O in the balanced equation is

    A. 1   B. 2   C. 3   D. 4   E. 5

21. For the reaction $Fe + O_2 \rightarrow Fe_2O_3$, the coefficient that would appear in front of Fe in the balanced equation is

    A. 1   B. 2   C. 3   D. 4   E. 5

22. For the reaction $PbS + O_2 \rightarrow PbO + SO_2$, the coefficient that would appear in front of Fe in the balanced equation is

    A. 1   B. 2   C. 3   D. 4   E. 5

23. For the reaction $C_2H_5OH + O_2 \rightarrow CO_2 + H_2O$, the coefficient that would appear in front of CO_2 in the balanced equation is

    A. 1   B. 2   C. 3   D. 4   E. 5

24. For the reaction of sulfur dioxide with oxygen, the coefficient that would appear in front of sulfur dioxide in the balanced equation is

    A. 1   B. 2   C. 3   D. 4   E. 5

25. The class of compound to which CH_3COOH belongs is

    A. acid   B. base   C. hydrocarbon
    D. alcohol   E. ether

KEY (CORRECT ANSWERS)

1. C
2. C
3. A
4. B
5. C

6. B
7. A
8. A
9. A
10. A

11. C
12. E
13. A
14. C
15. A

16. A
17. D
18. B
19. A
20. C

21. D
22. D
23. B
24. B
25. A

TEST 4

DIRECTIONS: Each question or incomplete statement is followed by several suggested answers or completions. Select the one that *BEST* answers the question or completes the statement. *PRINT THE LETTER OF THE CORRECT ANSWER IN THE SPACE AT THE RIGHT.*

1. An acid may be defined as a(n)   1.___

   A. electron donor
   B. proton acceptor
   C. hydrogen containing compound
   D. proton donor
   E. strong electrolyte

2. Hydrogen may be prepared by reacting a base with   2.___

   A. aluminum B. copper C. iron
   D. water   E. potassium chlorate

3. A piece of copper is coated with copper oxide.   3.___
   A substance that could be used to remove the oxide coating without affecting the copper is

   A. sodium hydroxide   B. calcium sulfate
   C. sodium carbonate   D. hydrochloric acid
   E. potassium nitrate

4. When acid is spilled, a common substance which could be used to neutralize the acid without producing harmful effects itself is   4.___

   A. sodium hydroxide   B. sodium bicarbonate
   C. sodium chloride   D. D, vinegar
   E. hydrogen chloride

5. A solution is classified as a mixture because   5.___

   A. it does not appear homogeneous
   B. the proportions of solute and solvent are variable
   C. it requires chemical methods to separate it into its various components
   D. all liquids are mixtures
   E. it may be saturated

6. The arrangement of the electrons for $_{11}Na^{23}$ can be expressed as   6.___

   A. $1s^2 2s^2 2p^6 3s^1$
   B. $1s^2 2s^2 2p^6 3s^2 3p^6 4s^2 4p^3$
   C. $1s^2 2s^2 2p^7$
   D. $1s^2 2s^8 3s^1$
   E. $1s^2 2s^8 3s^{13}$

7. The chemical atomic weight of chlorine of 35.5 can be accounted for by   7.___

   A. mass energy relations
   B. natural occurring chlorine being a mixture of two isotopes of chlorine

C. the mass of the electron being .5
D. the mass of the neutron being .5
E. the mass of the proton being .5

8. In phosphoric acid, the bond between phosphorus and the oxygen to which *no* hydrogen is attached is a(n) _____ bond.

   A. ionic
   B. coordinate covalent
   C. double
   D. ion dipole
   E. nonpolar covalent

9. A factor that will increase the rate of reaction between steel wool and oxygen is

   A. a decrease in temperature
   B. a decrease in surface area of the steel wool
   C. an increase in concentration of oxygen
   D. the presence of nitrogen
   E. the presence of Fe_2O_3

10. Isotopes of an element have

    A. the same number of electrons in the outermost shell
    B. the same atomic weight
    C. the same number of neutrons in the nucleus
    D. different number of protons in their nucleus
    E. different oxidation numbers

11. A tank for storing dilute sulfuric acid could be made from

    A. Fe   B. Al   C. Cu   D. Zn   E. Hg

12. A sample of temporary hard water is boiled. The precipitate is

    A. $Ca(HCO_3)_2$ B. $CaCO_3$ C. Na_2CO_3 D. NaCl   E. $CaSO_4$

13. Two clear liquids, when mixed with each other, yield a solid and a liquid. This represents

    A. precipitation
    B. condensation
    C. evaporation
    D. homogenization
    E. sublimation

14. One would predict that copper would react with nitric acid because

    A. copper is an active metal
    B. hydrogen would be formed
    C. nitric acid is a very strong oxidizing agent
    D. copper nitrate is insoluble
    E. nitric acid is a strong acid

15. One would predict that magnesium would react with hydrochloric acid, as

    A. magnesium chloride is insoluble
    B. water, a nonionized substance would be formed
    C. magnesium is above hydrogen in the activity series
    D. magnesium chloride, an ionized substance would form
    E. hydrochloric acid is a strong oxidizing agent

16. When magnesium oxide reacts with water

    A. hydrogen is evolved
    B. the hydroxide ion concentration of the solution is increased
    C. the hydrogen or hydronium ion concentration of the solution is increased
    D. hydrogen oxide is formed
    E. oxygen is evolved

17. When sulfur dioxide reacts with water,

    A. oxygen is evolved
    B. hydrogen is evolved
    C. the hydrogen or hydronium ion concentration of the solution is increased
    D. the hydroxide ion concentration of the solution is increased
    E. sulfur trioxide is formed

18. When zinc reacts with sulfuric acid,

    A. hydrogen is evolved
    B. oxygen is evolved
    C. water is formed
    D. the hydrogen ion concentration of the solution is increased
    E. zinc sulfate, an insoluble substance, is formed

19. When CH_4 reacts with oxygen,

    A. hydrogen is formed
    B. water is formed
    C. carbon monoxide, an ionic substance is formed
    D. matter is destroyed
    E. carbon dioxide precipitates

20. When calcium carbonate reacts with hydrochloric acid,

    A. carbon dioxide is evolved
    B. hydrogen is evolved
    C. oxygen is evolved
    D. calcium chloride precipitates
    E. moist pink litmus would be turned blue by the gas evolved

21. When ammonium chloride reacts with sodium hydroxide,

    A. hydrogen is evolved
    B. sodium chloride, an insoluble substance, forms
    C. hydrogen chloride is evolved
    D. moist pink litmus would be turned blue by the gas evolved
    E. the ammonium ion is formed

22. One would predict that silver nitrate should react with hydrochloric acid, as   22.____

   A. silver is an active metal
   B. silver chloride is insoluble
   C. hydrochloric acid, is an oxidizing agent
   D. hydrogen can be formed
   E. nitric acid, an oxidizing agent, can be formed

23. The chemical atomic weight of chlorine of 35.5 can be accounted for by   23.____

   A. natural occuring chlorine being a mixture of two isotopes of chlorine
   B. the mass of the electron being .5
   C. the mass of the proton being .5
   D. the mass of the neutron being .5
   E. mass energy relations

24. Isotopes of an element have   24.____

   A. the same atomic weight
   B. the same number of neutrons in the nucleus
   C. different oxidation numbers
   D. the same atomic numbers
   E. different numbers of protons in their nucleus

25. A tank for storing dilute hydrochloric acid could be made from   25.____

   A. copper   B. iron   C. aluminum
   D. mercury   E. zinc

KEY (CORRECT ANSWERS)

1.	D	11.	C
2.	A	12.	B
3.	D	13.	A
4.	B	14.	C
5.	B	15.	C
6.	A	16.	B
7.	B	17.	C
8.	B	18.	A
9.	C	19.	B
10.	A	20.	A

21. D
22. B
23. A
24. D
25. A

EXAMINATION SECTION
TEST 1

DIRECTIONS: Each question or incomplete statement is followed by several suggested answers or completions. Select the one that BEST answers the question or completes the statement. *PRINT THE LETTER OF THE CORRECT ANSWER IN THE SPACE AT THE RIGHT.*

1. The molecular weight of magnesium acetate, $Mg(C_2H_3O_2)_2$, is   1._____

    A. 15   B. 16   C. 83   D. 142   E. 166

2. Which class of compounds would give *only* carbon dioxide and water on complete combustion?   2._____

    A. Salts   B. Bases   C. Proteins
    D. Hydrocarbons   E. Basic oxides

3. A molecule is said to be polar if it   3._____

    A. has a north and south pole
    B. has a symmetrical electron distribution
    C. exhibits a polar spin under certain conditions
    D. may exhibit a positive or negative charge
    E. exhibits a partial positive charge at one end and a partial negative charge at the other

4. In the reaction represented by $MnO_2 + 4HCl \rightarrow MnCl_2 + 2H_2O + Cl_2$, the oxidation number of manganese has   4._____

    A. *decreased* from 0 to -2
    B. *decreased* from +4 to +2
    C. *remained* the same
    D. *increased* from +1 to +2
    E. *increased* from -2 to +4

5. When an atom of a metal becomes an ion,   5._____

    A. it is reduced
    B. it gains protons
    C. it gains electrons
    D. the ionic radius becomes less than the atomic radius
    E. the ionic radius becomes greater than the atomic radius

6. Ethyl benzene, $C_6H_5 - C_2H_5$, and dimethyl benzene, $C_6H_4(CH_3)_2$, are examples of   6._____

    A. isomers   B. isotopes
    C. allotropes   D. homogeneous mixtures
    E. heterogeneous mixtures

7. Each atom of any of the elements in Group IA has one electron in its outermost shell. The element in which the electron is held LEAST securely is   7._____

    A. the strongest reducing agent
    B. the smallest in diameter
    C. the strongest electron acceptor
    D. the least active of the group
    E. located in the middle of the group

8. The number of neutrons in the nucleus of an atom of $_4Be^9$ is

    A. 36   B. 13   C. 9   D. 4   E. 5

9. As acetic acid is slowly added to a solution of ammonium hydroxide, the conductivity INCREASES because

    A. a soluble compound is formed
    B. acetic acid dissociates readily
    C. the pH of the solution is changed
    D. the ion concentration increases
    E. neutralization is an exothermic reaction

10. If two isotopes of a certain element are known, it follows that the atoms of that element

    A. are radioactive
    B. differ chemically from each other
    C. have different numbers of protons in their nuclei
    D. have different numbers of neutrons in their nuclei
    E. have different numbers of electrons surrounding their nuclei

11. The density of oxygen at STP may be obtained from

    A. $\dfrac{16 \text{ grams}}{22.4 \text{ liters}}$
    B. $\dfrac{22.4 \text{ grams}}{16 \text{ liters}}$
    C. $\dfrac{32 \text{ grams}}{22.4 \text{ liters}}$
    D. $\dfrac{22.4 \text{ grams}}{32 \text{ liters}}$
    E. $\dfrac{22.4 \text{ grams}}{11.2 \text{ liters}}$

12. Twenty milliliters of chlorine gas and fifty milliliters of hydrogen gas were mixed at STP and reacted.
    When the products were returned to STP, the amount of unreacted gas was _____ milliliters.

    A. 10   B. 20   C. 25   D. 30   E. 50

13. Which of these has a zero rest mass?

    A. Alpha particle   B. Proton   C. Neutron
    D. Beta ray   E. Gamma ray

14. The nucleus of an isotope of tin, $_{50}Sn^{116}$, contains

    A. 50 neutrons
    B. 50 protons
    C. 66 electrons
    D. 116 protons
    E. 166 total of protons plus neutrons

15. A vessel contains 2.50 moles of oxygen gas, 0.50 mole of nitrogen gas, and 1.00 mole of carbon dioxide gas. The total pressure is 2.00 atmospheres.
    The partial pressure exerted by the oxygen in the mixture is _____ atmospheres.

    A. 1.25   B. 1.50   C. 1.66   D. 2.00   E. 2.50

16. If one mole of an acid neutralizes two moles of a base, then

    A. the acid is twice as concentrated as the base
    B. the base is twice as concentrated as the acid
    C. one mole of acid supplies one-half mole of hydrogen ions
    D. one mole of acid supplies one mole of hydrogen ions
    E. one mole of acid supplies two moles of hydrogen ions

17. A quantity of dry gas measures 254 milliliters at 27° C. When the temperature becomes 17° C at constant pressure, the gas measures _____ milliliters.

    A. $254 \times \frac{300}{290}$
    B. $254 \times \frac{290}{300}$
    C. $254 \times \frac{290}{246}$
    D. $254 \times \frac{300}{256}$
    E. $254 \times \frac{256}{273}$

18. In liquid water, the STRONGEST bonds between water molecules are _____ bonds.

    A. ionic
    B. covalent
    C. hydrogen
    D. van der Waals
    E. coordinate covalent

Questions 19-22.

DIRECTIONS: Use the following portion of the Periodic Table to answer Questions 19 through 22.

H							He
Li	Be	B	C	N	O	F	Ne
Na	Mg	Al	Si	P	S	Cl	Ar

19. The element requiring the LEAST amount of energy to remove one electron from an atom is

    A. Na   B. Be   C. O   D. Cl   E. Ar

20. One mole of which element will replace the GREATEST weight of hydrogen from dilute hydrochloric acid?

    A. Na   B. Mg   C. Al   D. S   E. Cl

21. The element whose atom shows the GREATEST affinity for an additional electron is

   A. H   B. He   C. N   D. Mg   E. F

22. The MOST active nonmetal in the period (row) starting with Na is

   A. Na   B. Mg   C. Si   D. Ar   E. Cl

23. Forty grams of helium at STP has a volume of _____ liters.

   A. 11.2   B. 22.4   C. 112   D. 224   E. 448

24. The oxidation number of cobalt in $Co(NH_3)_6Cl_3$ is

   A. +1   B. +2   C. +3   D. +4   E. +6

25. In a titration of H_2SO_4 with 5.0 N NaOH, 38 milliliters of the base was used to neutralize 95 milliliters of the acid.
The normality of the acid is

   A. $\dfrac{5.0\ N \times 38\ ml}{95\ ml}$ B. $\dfrac{5.0\ N \times 95\ ml}{38\ ml}$ C. $\dfrac{95\ ml}{5.0\ N \times 38\ ml}$

   D. $\dfrac{38\ ml \times 95\ ml}{5.0\ N}$ E. $5.0\ N \times 38\ ml \times 95\ ml$

26. Which of these gases measured under the same conditions of pressure and temperature has the GREATEST density?

   A. H_2 B. SO_2 C. NH_3 D. CH_4 E. CO_2

27. The characteristic of a compound that is CLOSELY related to its heat of formation is its

   A. density   B. stability   C. volatility
   D. solubility   E. boiling point

28. Sulfur dioxide gas and oxygen gas react in a closed system and form sulfur trioxide gas. The reaction is represented by the equation $2SO_2 + O_2 \rightleftarrows 2SO_3 + 44$ kilocalories.
The concentration of sulfur trioxide may be INCREASED by

   A. *decreasing* the pressure of the system at constant temperature
   B. *increasing* the pressure of the system at constant temperature
   C. *decreasing* the concentration of oxygen
   D. *increasing* the temperature of the system at constant pressure
   E. *decreasing* the concentration of sulfur dioxide

29. The gaseous molecules which have the GREATEST average velocity at 150°C are represented by

   A. O_2 B. F_2 C. H_2 D. N_2 E. H_2O

30. A sample of a compound contains 54.5 grams of carbon, 9.1 grams of hydrogen, and 36.4 grams of oxygen.
The SIMPLEST formula of this compound is

   A. CHO   B. C_2H_4O C. $C_4H_8O_2$ D. C_4H_8O E. C_5H_9O

31. The compound NOT properly named is

   A. Fe_2O_3, iron (III) oxide
   B. Pb_3O_4, trilead tetraoxide
   C. $CuCl_2$, copper (II) chloride
   D. $Pb_3(PO_4)_2$, lead (III) phosphate
   E. P_2S_5, diphosphorus pentasulfide

32. The general formula representing a ketone is

   A. R — OH
   B. $R-C\equiv N$
   C. R — O — R
   D. $R-\underset{\underset{O}{\|}}{C}-R$
   E. $R-\underset{\underset{O}{\|}}{C}-H$

33. Which compound is classed as a basic anhydride?

   A. BaO   B. SO_3 C. CO_2 D. NaOH   E. K_2CO_3

34. Copper oxide (CuO) reacts with hydrogen (H_2) and produces copper (Cu) and water (H_2O).
    How many moles of water can 240 grams of CuO produce? _____ moles.

    A. 1   B. 6   C. 3   D. 18   E. 54

35. What weight of solid sodium hydroxide is required to prepare 2.00 liters of a 3.00 molar solution? _____ grams.

    A. 40   B. 80   C. 240   D. 480   E. 667

36. The number of molecules present in 22.0 grams of carbon dioxide at STP is

   A. 2.01×10^{12}
   B. 6.03×10^{12}
   C. 2.06×10^{22}
   D. 3.01×10^{23}
   E. 6.02×10^{23}

37. In order for two electrons to occupy the same orbital, they must

   A. have opposite spins
   B. be oppositely charged
   C. enter the orbital simultaneously
   D. have the same spin value
   E. remain at constant distance from the center of the mass

38. When a concentrated solution of NaCl in water is electro-lyzed by a direct current using platinum electrodes, the products are

   A. H_2, Cl_2, and NaOH
   B. Cl_2O, H_2, and Na
   C. O_2, Cl_2, and Na
   D. H_2, HCl, and NaOH
   E. H_2, O_2, Cl_2, and Na

39. The density of a gas at 27° C and standard pressure is

   A. greater than at STP
   B. the same as at STP
   C. less than at STP
   D. greater than at standard pressure and 273° K
   E. less than at 310° K and standard pressure

40. In the reaction $P_4O_{10} + 6H_2O \rightarrow 4H_3PO_4$, the part played by the oxide of phosphorus is that of a(n)

   A. catalyst
   B. reducing agent
   C. basic anhydride
   D. oxidizing agent
   E. acid anhydride

41. A crystal of sodium chloride when added to a solution of sodium chloride that is in equilibrium with excess solid sodium chloride will

   A. dissolve in the solution
   B. form a supersaturated solution
   C. react with the water in the solution
   D. cause additional sodium chloride crystals to separate from the solution
   E. cause no visible change in the solution

42. Assuming complete ionization, the pH of a 0.01 M HCl solution would be

   A. 1   B. 2   C. 3   D. 4   E. 0.5

43. The boiling point of a one molal solution of a nonvolatile, nonelectrolyte is 100.52° C. The boiling point of a solution containing 90 grams of a nonvolatile, nonionizing compound dissolved in 1000 grams of water was found to be 100.78° C.
The APPROXIMATE molecular weight of the compound is

   A. 30   B. 60   C. 90   D. 135   E. 180

44. The same quantity of electricity is passed through a one molar solution of HCl and a one molar solution of H_2SO_4. The weight of hydrogen evolved from the H_2SO_4 as compared to that from the HCl is

   A. the same
   B. twice as much
   C. one-half as much
   D. dependent on the temperature
   E. dependent on the concentration

45. The APPROXIMATE number of molecules of hydrogen in 1.00 liter of H_2 gas at STP is

   A. 1.35×10^{22} B. 3.01×10^{23} C. 6.02×10^{23}
   D. 2.69×10^{22} E. 5.38×10^{22}

KEY (CORRECT ANSWERS)

1. D	11. C	21. E	31. D	41. E
2. D	12. D	22. E	32. D	42. B
3. E	13. E	23. D	33. A	43. B
4. B	14. B	24. C	34. C	44. A
5. D	15. A	25. A	35. C	45. D
6. A	16. E	26. B	36. D	
7. A	17. B	27. B	37. A	
8. E	18. C	28. B	38. A	
9. D	19. A	29. C	39. C	
10. D	20. C	30. B	40. E	

TEST 2

DIRECTIONS: Each question or incomplete statement is followed by several suggested answers or completions. Select the one that BEST answers the question or completes the statement. *PRINT THE LETTER OF THE CORRECT ANSWER IN THE SPACE AT THE RIGHT.*

1. A certain element designated as Y has an oxidation number of -3, and another element designated as X has an oxidation number of +2.
   The CORRECT formula for a chemical compound of the two elements is represented by

   A. XY   B. XY_2 C. X_2Y D. X_2Y_3 E. X_3Y_2

   1.____

2. If the table of atomic weights were established with the oxygen atom assigned the value of 100, then the atomic weight of a carbon atom would be APPROXIMATELY

   A. 12.0   B. 24.0   C. 37.5   D. 75.0   E. 112.0

   2.____

3. The total number of atoms represented by $5Al(C_2H_3O_2)_3$ is

   A. 22   B. 60   C. 71   D. 84   E. 110

   3.____

4. All of the oxygen is removed from a sample of $NaClO_3$ by heating.
   The BEST solvent for the residue is

   A. water   B. aqua regia
   C. nitric acid   D. carbon disulfide
   E. carbon tetrachloride

   4.____

5. A particle containing 5 protons, 4 electrons, and 6 neutrons weighs APPROXIMATELY as much as

   A. 10 protons   B. 11 neutrons   C. 15 neutrons
   D. 4 electrons   E. 5 protons

   5.____

6. Zn, Fe, and Cu are listed in order of decreasing reactivity.
   Which statement is CORRECT?

   A. Cu displaces both Zn^{++} and Fe^{++}.
   B. Zn displaces Cu^{++} but not Fe^{++}.
   C. Fe displaces Zn^{++} but not Cu^{++}.
   D. Cu displaces neither Zn^{++} nor Fe^{++}.
   E. Zn displaces neither Cu^{++} nor Fe^{++}.

   6.____

7. The number of neutrons in an atom of an element is

   A. the same in each isotope
   B. the same as the atomic number
   C. equal to the number of electrons
   D. equal to the number of protons in the nucleus
   E. equal to the difference between the mass number and the atomic number

   7.____

8. In BaCl$_2 \cdot$ 2H$_2$O, the water is

    A. absorbed from the air
    B. in ionization equilibrium
    C. mechanically held in the crystal
    D. referred to as water of crystallization
    E. referred to as water of ionization

9. The number of equivalent weights of solute per liter of solution is known as its

    A. molarity
    B. normality
    C. molality
    D. formality
    E. weight - percentage

10. The percentage of nitrogen in NH$_4$NO$_3$ is

    A. 17.5% B. 22.2% C. 28.0% D. 35.0% E. 57.5%

11. The salt water solution that tests NEAREST to 7 on the pH scale is

    A. NaCl B. NaHSO$_3$ C. NaHSO$_4$ D. NaHCO$_3$ E. Na$_2$CO$_3$

12. At a constant temperature in a saturated aqueous salt solution in contact with undissolved salt,

    A. addition of a common ion enables more salt to dissolve
    B. the rate of dissolving exceeds that of crystallization
    C. the rate of dissolving equals the rate of crystallization of the salt
    D. the weight of salt in solution equals the weight of undissolved salt
    E. all of the salt is found in the undissolved salt at the bottom of the container

13. The COMPLETE combustion of ethane in oxygen is represented by

    A. 2C$_2$H$_6$ + 7O$_2 \rightarrow$ 4CO$_2$ + 3H$_2$O
    B. 2C$_2$H$_6$ + 7O$_2 \rightarrow$ 4CO$_2$ + 6H$_2$O
    C. 2C$_2$H$_6$ + 5O$_2 \rightarrow$ 4CO + H$_2$O
    D. C$_2$H$_6$ + O$_2 \rightarrow$ 2CO + 3H$_2$
    E. C$_2$H$_6$ + 2O$_2 \rightarrow$ 2CO$_2$ + 3H$_2$

14. A chemical bond is considered to be predominantly ionic if

    A. atoms of the same element combine
    B. the reaction forming the bond is endothermic
    C. atoms of an active metal combine with the atoms of an active nonmetal
    D. the bond is between atoms of elements which are of the same family
    E. atoms of one metal combine with atoms of another metal

15. In the reaction represented by the equation
    3BaCl$_2$ + Fe$_2$(SO$_4$)$_3 \rightarrow$ 3BaSO$_4$ + 2FeCl$_3$, the products are favored because

    A. a soluble product forms
    B. one stable product forms
    C. a slightly soluble product forms
    D. the reaction is reversible
    E. a volatile product escapes

16. The functional group characteristic of organic acids is

A. O
    ‖
    — C — OH

B. O
    ‖
    — C — H

C. O
    ‖
    — C — R

D. — O — R

E. — C ≡ N

17. Element X forms an oxide whose formula is X_2O_3.
    The group to which element X belongs in the Periodic Table is MOST likely Group

    A. IA   B. IIA   C. IIIA   D. VIA   E. VIIA

Questions 18-20.

DIRECTIONS: Use the following portion of the Periodic Table to answer Questions 18 through 20.

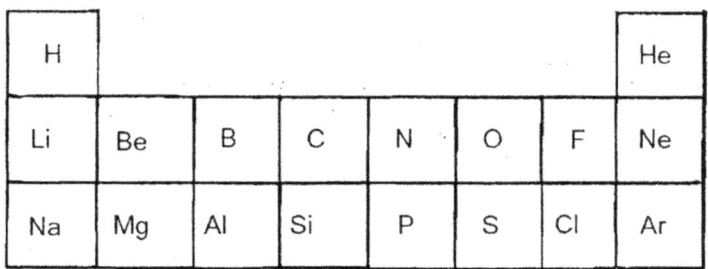

18. The number of valence electrons in the outermost shell of O is

    A. 8   B. 2   C. 3   D. 6   E. 5

19. The MOST probable oxidation number of Al in a compound is

    A. -4   B. +3   C. +4   D. +5   E. +7

20. The element MOST likely to form covalent compounds is

    A. Li   B. Be   C. C   D. F   E. Ar

21. Which equation represents the reaction of hot carbon with steam?

    A. $C + H_2O \rightarrow CO + H_2$
    B. $C + 2H_2O \rightarrow CO_2 + 2H_2$
    C. $2C + 6H_2O \rightarrow 2H_2CO_3 + 4H_2$
    D. $C + 2H_2O \rightarrow C + 2H_2 + O_2$
    E. $C + H_2O \rightarrow H_2CO$

22. The half life of Po^{210} is 140 days.   22._____
Starting with 2.00 grams of Po^{210}, how much will be left after 280 days? _____
gram(s).

   A. 0.25　　B. 0.50　　C. 1.00　　D. 1.25　　E. 1.50

23. According to the Avogadro Principle, one liter of gaseous hydrogen and one liter of gaseous ammonia contain the SAME number of   23._____

   A. atoms at standard conditions
   B. molecules at all conditions
   C. molecules only at standard conditions
   D. atoms if conditions in both containers are the same
   E. molecules if conditions in both containers are the same

24. The weight of one liter at CO$_2$ at STP is_____ grams.   24._____

   A. 1.96　　B. 2.00　　C. 12.0　　D. 28.0　　E. 44.0

25. One liter of oxygen is collected by displacement of water. The barometric pressure, corrected for vapor pressure, is 782 millimeters of mercury, and the room temperature is 21° C.   25._____
The volume of oxygen at STP is _____ milliliters.

   A. $1000 \times \frac{782}{760} \times \frac{273}{294}$　　B. $1000 \times \frac{760}{782} \times \frac{273}{294}$　　C. $1000 \times \frac{782}{760} \times \frac{294}{273}$

   D. $1000 \times \frac{782}{760} \times \frac{21}{0}$　　E. $1000 \times \frac{273}{760} \times \frac{294}{782}$

26. The molecular weight of a compound is 75. A student reported an experimental value of 78.   26._____
His percent error is

   A. $\frac{(78-75)}{78}$　　B. $\frac{75}{78} \times 100$　　C. $\frac{78}{75} \times 100$

   D. $\frac{(78-75)}{75} \times 100$　　E. $\frac{(78-75)}{78} \times 100$

27. Fluorine is the MOST active halogen principally because among the halogens, it has the   27._____

   A. *fastest* molecules
   B. *smallest* atomic radius
   C. *lowest* density
   D. *lowest* boiling point
   E. *smallest* number of neutrons

28. A 500 milliliter sample of gas at STP weighs 0.581 grams. The composition of gas is C = 92.24% and H = 7.76%.   28._____
The molecular formula of the gas is

   A. CH_4　　B. C_2H_2　　C. C_2H_4　　D. C_3H_6　　E. C_4H_{10}

29. To neutralize 75 milliliters of hydrochloric acid requires 25 milliliters of 3 molar sodium hydroxide. The hydrochloric acid is

    A. 1 molal   B. 2 normal   C. 3 normal
    D. 1 molar   E. 3 molar

30. According to their heats of formation, the MOST stable of these compounds is _____ kilocalories per mole.

    A. HI −5.9   B. H_2S +5.3   C. HBr +8.6
    D. HCl +22.0   E. HF + 64.2

31. When two grams of carbon are burned to carbon dioxide, 15.75 kilocalories of heat energy are liberated.
The heat liberated during the formation of one mole of carbon dioxide is _____ kilocalories per mole.

    A. 15.75   B. 31.50   C. 47.25   D. 63.00   E. 94.50

32. $H_2O + CO_3^{--}$ $HCO_3^- + OH^-$
According to the Bronsted-Lowry concept of acid-base reactions, the acids in the equation written above are

    A. H_2O and OH^- B. HCO_3^- and OH^- C. H_2O and HCO_3^-
    D. CO_3^{--} and HCO_3^- E. H_2O and CO_3^{--}

33. The CORRECT electronic configuration for the sodium atom, $_{11}Na^{23}$, is

    A. $1s^2 2s^2 2p^6$ B. $1s^2 2s^2 2p^6 3s^1$
    C. $1s^2 2s^2 2p^4 3s^2 3p^1$ D. $1s^2 2s^2 2p^8 2d^{10} 3s^1$
    E. $1s^2 2s^2 2p^6 2d^{10} 3s^2 3p^1$

34. In electrolysis, the reaction at the anode is called

    A. ionization   B. hydrolysis   C. oxidation
    D. reduction   E. neutralization

35. A sample of carbon dioxide at STP weighs 11 grams. The weight of the same number of molecules of sulfur dioxide at STP is _____ grams.

    A. 4   B. 8   C. 16   D. 32   E. 64

36. Assuming that the reaction $N_2 + 3H_2 \rightarrow 2NH_3$ uses up all reactants, the volume of nitrogen necessary to form 400 liters of ammonia at the same temperature and pressure is _____ liters of N_2.

    A. 100   B. 200   C. 300   D. 400   E. 600

37. One liter of a gas weighs 1.25 grams at STP. The gas

    A. is diatomic
    B. is easily liquefied
    C. has a molecular weight of 28
    D. has a greater density than air
    E. is 1.25 times as heavy as a liter of hydrogen

38. A molecule of deuterium oxide differs from an ordinary water molecule because deuterium oxide has

    A. two atoms of oxygen
    B. three atoms of hydrogen
    C. a positive or negative charge
    D. oxygen atoms of atomic mass 17
    E. hydrogen atoms of atomic mass 2

39. The oxidation number of carbon s minus two (-2) in

    A. CO   B. CCl_4 C. $CHCl_3$ D. CH_2Cl_2 E. CH_3Cl

40. An atom and an ion of the same element have the same

    A. color
    B. nuclear charge
    C. electronic charge
    D. chemical properties
    E. physical properties

41. An explanation of the heat of vaporization of water being much higher than the heat of vaporization of ethane (C_2H_6) is that

    A. ethane has dipole molecules
    B. water is denser than liquid ethane
    C. water has a higher boiling point than ethane
    D. water molecules are lighter than ethane molecules
    E. energy is needed to break the hydrogen bonding between water molecules

42. The number of grams of oxygen in 1.5 moles of oxygen is _____ grams.

    A. 12   B. 16   C. 24   D. 32   E. 48

43. In the reaction, represented by the equation
    $2As + 3NaOH \rightarrow Na_3AsO_3 + AsH_3$, the volume at STP of arsine gas (AsH_3) produced from 25 grams of arsenic is _____ liters.

    A. 3.7   B. 7.5   C. 11.2   D. 14.7   E. 22.4

44. The freezing point of a molal solution of a nonelectrolyte is -1.86° C if the solvent is water.
    The freezing point of a molal solution of $CaCl_2$, assuming complete ionization and neglecting interionic attraction, would be

    A. 0.00° C   B. -1.86° C   C. -3.72° C   D. -5.58° C   E. -9.93° C

45. Assuming that one liter of HCl solution contains two times the Avogadro number of ions, the molarity of the solution is

    A. 1.0   B. 2.0   C. 3.0   D. 6.0   E. 0.5

KEY (CORRECT ANSWERS)

1. E	11. A	21. A	31. E	41. E
2. D	12. C	22. B	32. C	42. E
3. E	13. B	23. E	33. B	43. A
4. A	14. C	24. A	34. C	44. D
5. B	15. C	25. A	35. C	45. A
6. D	16. A	26. D	36. B	
7. E	17. C	27. B	37. C	
8. D	18. D	28. B	38. E	
9. B	19. B	29. D	39. E	
10. D	20. C	30. E	40. B	

EXAMINATION SECTION
TEST 1

DIRECTIONS: Each question or incomplete statement is followed by several suggested answers or completions. Select the one that BEST answers the question or completes the statement. *PRINT THE LETTER OF THE CORRECT ANSWER IN THE SPACE AT THE RIGHT.*

The following list of atomic weights may be referred to in solving problems involving computations:

Aluminum	27.0	Hydrogen	1.0	Phosphorous	31.0
Bromine	79.9	Iodine	126.9	Silver	107.9
Calcium	40.1	Iron	55.9	Sodium	23.0
Carbon	12.0	Lead	207.2	Sulfur	32.0
Chlorine	35.5	Nitrogen	14.0	Tin	118.7
Copper	63.5	Oxygen	16.0	Zinc	65.4

1. A solution of 0.02 M HCl has a pH of

    A. 1.7   B. 2.0   C. 2.3   D. 2.7

2. The pH of a saturated solution of CO_2 in water at 25 °C is MOST NEARLY

    A. 3   B. 5   C. 7   D. 9

3. An aqueous solution containing 100 grams of HCl per liter of solution is APPROXIMATELY _____ N.

    A. 1.0   B. 2.8   C. 3.2   D. 12.0

4. The volume of 12 N HCl which must be taken and made up to 100 ml with distilled water in order to make 100 ml of 1 N HCl is _____ ml.

    A. 1.2   B. 6.5   C. 8.3   D. 12

5. Of the following, the one which has the HIGHEST melting point is

    A. benzoic acid
    B. lead
    C. sodium chloride
    D. sulfur

6. Of the following, the one which has the LOWEST boiling point is

    A. $CH_3\text{-}CH_3$
    B. $CH_3\text{-}CO\text{-}CH_3$
    C. $CH_3\text{-}CH_2\text{-}O\text{-}CH_2\text{-}CH_3$
    D. CCl_4

7. Of the following, the one which has the HIGHEST boiling point is

    A. CH_3COOH B. HCl   C. HNO_3 D. H_2SO_4

8. Of the following, the STRONGEST oxidizing agent is

    A. $CrCl_3$ B. I_2 C. $KMnO_4$ D. $SnCl_2$

9. Of the following, the STRONGEST reducing agent is

    A. $BaCl_2$ B. $FeCl_3$ C. $Na_2S_2O_3$ D. $Na_2S_4O_6$

10. Of the following substances, the one with the HIGHEST softening point is 10._____

    A. Pyrex   B. quartz
    C. soda-lime glass   D. Vycor

11. The purpose of annealing glass is to 11._____

    A. give a shiny finish   B. increase the ductility
    C. relieve strains   D. remove fogging

12. Of the following reagents, the one which is NOT corrosive to chemical glassware is hot 12._____

    A. 12 M HCl
    B. 16 M HNO_3
    C. conc. HCl + conc. HNO_3
    D. saturated NaOH

13. Of the following reagents, the one which is MOST corrosive to a platinum crucible is 13._____

    A. a mixture of conc. HCl and conc. HNO_3
    B. boiling H_2SO_4
    C. fused NaOH
    D. hot 12 M NH_3

14. Of the following metals, the one which is MOST active chemically is 14._____

    A. copper   B. iron   C. mercury   D. zinc

15. Of the following gases, the one which is MOST soluble in water is 15._____

    A. CO_2 B. HCl   C. H_2S D. N_2

16. Of the following, the gas with the GREATEST density at standard temperature and pressure is 16._____

    A. air   B. carbon dioxide
    C. hydrogen sulfide   D. methane

17. Water is at its GREATEST density at a temperature of 17._____

    A. 0° C   B. 4° C   C. 20° C   D. 37° C

18. The term Ostwald refers to a type of apparatus GENERALLY used to determine 18._____

    A. color   B. refractive index
    C. temperature   D. viscosity

19. The term Beilstein refers to a chemical 19._____

    A. reference book   B. society
    C. technique   D. unit of radioactivity

20. The term Westphal refers to a type of apparatus GENERALLY used to determine 20._____

    A. boiling point elevation B. freezing point
    C. refractive index   D. specific gravity

21. The recommended solder for ordinary electrical connections is

    A. Babbitt metal
    B. resin-core solder
    C. silver solder
    D. soft solder with an acid flux

22. Soft solder is composed PRINCIPALLY of lead and

    A. antimony   B. bismuth   C. cadmium   D. tin

23. Solid Na_2CO_3 is BEST removed from a saturated solution of NaOH by

    A. distillation
    B. filtration through ashless filter paper
    C. filtration through a Gooch crucible with asbestos
    D. filtration through a sintered glass funnel

24. A Type K potentiometer is USUALLY used for measuring

    A. amount of electrical charge
    B. parachor
    C. refractive index
    D. voltage

25. A Wheatstone bridge is FREQUENTLY used to

    A. calibrate photographic developer
    B. determine optical rotation
    C. measure electrical resistance
    D. support electrodes

26. The McLeod gauge is used to measure

    A. amperage   B. humidity
    C. low pressures   D. low temperatures

27. The minimum amount of liquid needed for an accurate pyknometric determination of its density is MOST NEARLY

    A. 0.1 liter   B. 1.0 liter
    C. 0.1 ml   D. 10 ml

28. The minimum volume of liquid needed for routine measurement of its refractive index is MOST NEARLY _____ ml.

    A. 0.1   B. 1.0   C. 10   D. 100

29. Of the following, the one which is NOT intended for measuring temperature is the

    A. iron-contstantan thermocouple
    B. mercury thermoregulator
    C. nickel resistance thermometer
    D. optical pyrometer

30. The only one of the following substances which is SAFE to heat is

    A. ammonium nitrate
    B. lead azide
    C. perchloric acid
    D. potassium persulfate

31. The PRINCIPAL function of the *fix* in photographic processing is to

    A. dissolve the unreacted gelatine
    B. dissolve the unreacted silver
    C. dissolve the unreacted silver halide
    D. tan the emulsion

32. The temperature of an incandescent object which is glowing cherry red is APPROXIMATELY _____ °C.

    A. 250   B. 400   C. 700   D. 1300

33. Chromatography is used PRINCIPALLY for

    A. carbon and hydrogen analysis of organic compounds
    B. purification of industrial water supplies
    C. quantitative inorganic analysis
    D. separation of small amounts of organic compounds from mixtures

34. A unit of radioactivity is the

    A. microcurie
    B. microlumen
    C. microradian
    D. microwave

35. Of the following substances, the one with the LOWEST solubility in water (measured in grams per liter) is

    A. barium chloride
    B. calcium nitrate
    C. ferrous sulfate
    D. mercurous chloride

36. The solubility product of AgCl is 10^{-10}.
    The solubility of AgCl in a 0.1 M NaCl solution is MOST NEARLY _____ moles/liter.

    A. 10^{-11} B. 10^{-9} C. 10^{-5} D. 10^{-1}

37. A violet color in a flame test indicates the presence of

    A. lithium   B. potassium   C. sodium   D. strontium

38. The one of the following which will dissolve 10 gms of AgI is 100 ml of

    A. 1 M HNO_3 B. 1 M NH^3 C. 6 M HCl   D. 6 M NaCN

39. The one of the following substances which is NOT white is

    A. aluminum hydroxide
    B. cuprous chloride
    C. mercuric iodide
    D. zinc sulfate

40. An unknown white solid dissolves in 6 M NH_3 to give a clear colorless solution. It, therefore, CANNOT contain _____ ions.

    A. magnesium   B. mercuric   C. silver   D. zinc

KEY (CORRECT ANSWERS)

1. A	11. C	21. B	31. C
2. B	12. D	22. D	32. C
3. B	13. A	23. C	33. D
4. C	14. D	24. D	34. A
5. C	15. B	25. C	35. D
6. A	16. B	26. C	36. B
7. D	17. B	27. D	37. B
8. C	18. D	28. A	38. D
9. C	19. A	29. B	39. C
10. B	20. D	30. D	40. B

TEST 2

DIRECTIONS: Each question or incomplete statement is followed by several suggested answers or completions. Select the one that BEST answers the question or completes the statement. *PRINT THE LETTER OF THE CORRECT ANSWER IN THE SPACE AT THE RIGHT.*

1. In titrating 0.1 M acetic acid with 0.1 M NaOH, the CORRECT endpoint will be at a pH of APPROXIMATELY   1._____

    A. 2 B. 5 C. 9 D. 11

2. Potassium thiocyanate gives a reddish color with aqueous solutions of _____ ions.   2._____

    A. cuprous B. ferric C. lead D. magnesium

3. Of the following, the one used in the colorimetric test for low concentrations of ammonia in water is   3._____

    A. Fehling's Solution
    B. Karl Fischer Reagent
    C. Nessler Reagent
    D. Ringer's Solution

4. Dimethylglyoxime is a reagent used to detect the presence of   4._____

    A. chlorine B. lead C. nickel D. tin

5. In the gravimetric analysis of a chloride, the weighing form is NORMALLY   5._____

    A. AgCl B. $BaCl_2$ C. Hg_2Cl_2 D. NaCl

6. Of the following salts, the one which is MOST soluble in water at room temperature is   6._____

    A. Ag_2SO_4 B. $BaSO_4$ C. CaC_2O_4 D. $MgSO_4$

7. The one of the following solids which is MOST soluble in 8 M NaOH is   7._____

    A. $BaSO_4$
    B. $Fe(OH)_3$
    C. hydrated aluminum hydroxide
    D. hydrated silver hydroxide

8. Of the following, the one which is the amide group is   8._____

    A. $-\overset{O}{\overset{\|}{C}}-NH_2$ B. $-N\overset{CH_3}{\underset{CH_3}{\diagup\!\!\!\diagdown}}$ C. $-NH_2$ D. $-N=O$

9. The linkage between the amino acid units of a protein is called   9._____

    A. ether linkage
    B. hydrogen bond
    C. oxazole linkage
    D. peptide linkage

10. Of the following compounds, the one which will react MOST vigorously with sodium at room temperature is   10._____

318

A. CH_3CH_2OH

B. $CH_3-\underset{\underset{O}{\|}}{C}-O-CH_3$

C. $CH_3CH_2-O-CH_2CH_3$

D. (benzene ring)

11. Of the following compounds, the one which possesses geometrical isomers is

    A. $CCl_2=CCl_2$ B. $CH_2=CCl_2$ C. $CH_2=CHCl$ D. $CHCl=CHCl$

12. Of the following, the one which is the STRONGEST acid is

    A. CCl_3COOH B. $CHCl_2COOH$ C. $CH_2ClCOOH$ D. CH_3COOH

13. Glucose is a
   A. disaccharide
   B. monosaccharide
   C. polysaccharide
   D. starch

14. Of the following, the one which is an example of an amino acid is
   A. cellulose   B. diastase   C. maltose   D. tyrosine

15. Of the following acids, the one with the LARGEST acid constant is
   A. acetic acid
   B. carbonic acid
   C. hydrocyanic acid
   D. hydrogen sulfide

16. A water solution of calcium oxide is
   A. acid   B. alkaline   C. neutral   D. a base

17. A water solution of aluminum chloride is
   A. acid   B. alkaline   C. neutral   D. a base

18. The vapor pressure of mercury at room temperature is APPROXIMATELY _____ mm Hg.
   A. 10^{-6} B. 10^{-3} C. 1   D. 760

19. Of the following elements, the ONLY one which is ferromagnetic is
   A. aluminum   B. boron   C. nickel   D. tungsten

20. Mixing gelatine with water gives a(n)
   A. emulsion
   B. lyophilic colloid
   C. lyophobic colloid
   D. suspension

21. In the reaction $Ra_{226}^{90} \rightarrow Th_{222}^{88} + X$, X is a(n)
   A. alpha particle
   B. beta particle
   C. gamma ray
   D. meson

22. Of the following, the one with the LEAST mass is the

    A. deuteron   B. electron   C. neutron   D. proton

23. Beer's law refers to the

    A. absorption of light in solutions
    B. boiling point of non-associated liquids
    C. surface tension of a homologous series of fatty acids
    D. vapor pressure of binary liquid mixtures

24. A spectrophotometer working in the ultraviolet and visible regions of the spectrum is PARTICULARLY useful in

    A. colorimetric analysis
    B. distinguishing the components of gasoline
    C. distinguishing optical isomers
    D. qualitative analysis of inorganic salts

25. The addition of a neutron to a nucleus

    A. raises the atomic number by one without changing the atomic weight
    B. raises the atomic weight by one without changing atomic weight
    C. raises both the atomic number and the atomic weight by one
    D. always causes nuclear fission to occur

26. Of the following elements, the only one which CANNOT be tested for on an emission spectrograph is

    A. copper   B. iron   C. mercury   D. oxygen

27. A gas which is LIGHTER than air has the formula

    A. C_2H_2 B. C_2H_6 C. N_2O D. NO_2

28. The kinetic theory of gases predicts that the viscosity of gases will _____ density.

    A. decrease with decreased
    B. vary with the square root of the
    C. increase with decreased
    D. be independent of

29. The specific resistance of a 0.1 N NaCl solution was found to be 93.6 ohms at 25°C. Its SPECIFIC conductance will be _____ ohms.

    A. 0.936
    B. 6.4 reciprocal
    C. 0.011 reciprocal
    D. 93.6

30. Pure carbon monoxide may be prepared in the laboratory by

    A. adding dilute sulfuric acid to marble chips
    B. adding concentrated sulfuric acid to formic acid
    C. burning coke in a limited supply of air
    D. adding dilute hydrochloric acid to limestone

31. Pound for pound, sodium carbonate, when compared with sodium bicarbonate, will provide _____ sodium ions and _____ carbon dioxide.
    A. fewer; less
    B. more; less
    C. more; more
    D. fewer; more

32. Water gas (synthesis gas) is MAINLY a mixture of
    A. CO and N_2
    B. CO and H_2
    C. CO_2 and H_2O
    D. CO and O_2

33. The anhydride of nitrous acid is
    A. NO
    B. N_2O_3
    C. N_2O_5
    D. NO_2

34. The percent of gold in 14-carat gold is APPROXIMATELY
    A. 58
    B. 78
    C. 83
    D. 70

35. Three of the following are ores of iron. The one which is NOT is
    A. siderite
    B. hematite
    C. limonite
    D. spiegeleisen

36. The symbol of the element with the GREATEST tendency to gain electrons is
    A. F
    B. Bi
    C. At
    D. O

37. The Kroll process is used for extracting
    A. geramium
    B. molybdenum
    C. titanium
    D. wolfram

38. Waste rock material in an ore is called
    A. gangue
    B. slag
    C. flux
    D. iroth

39. Cementite is of fundamental importance in iron alloys. Its formula is
    A. FeC
    B. Fe_2C
    C. Fe_3C
    D. Fe_4C_3

40. Lead is dissolved MOST readily in dilute _____ acid.
    A. acetic
    B. sulfuric
    C. hydrochloric
    D. phosphoric

KEY (CORRECT ANSWERS)

1. C	11. D	21. A	31. D
2. B	12. A	22. B	32. A
3. C	13. B	23. A	33. A
4. C	14. D	24. A	34. B
5. A	15. A	25. D	35. C
6. D	16. B	26. D	36. A
7. C	17. A	27. A	37. B
8. A	18. B	28. C	38. A
9. D	19. C	29. A	39. A
10. A	20. B	30. D	40. A

SCIENCE READING COMPREHENSION
EXAMINATION SECTION
TEST 1

DIRECTIONS: Each question or incomplete statement is followed by several suggested answers or completions. Select the one that BEST answers the question or completes the statement. *PRINT THE LETTER OF THE CORRECT ANSWER IN THE SPACE AT THE RIGHT.*

PASSAGE

Photosynthesis is a complex process with many intermediate steps. Ideas differ greatly as to the details of these steps, but the general nature of the process and its outcome are well established. Water, usually from the soil, is conducted through the xylem of root, stem and leaf to the chlorophyl-containing cells of a leaf. In consequence of the abundance of water within the latter cells, their walls are saturated with water. Carbon dioxide, diffusing from the air through the stomata and into the intercellular spaces of the leaf, comes into contact with the water in the walls of the cells which adjoin the intercellular spaces. The carbon dioxide becomes dissolved in the water of these walls, and in solution diffuses through the walls and the plasma membranes into the cells. By the agency of chlorophyl in the chloroplasts of the cells, the energy of light is transformed into chemical energy. This chemical energy is used to decompose the carbon dioxide and water, and the products of their decomposition are recombined into a new compound. The compound first formed is successively built up into more and more complex substances until finally a sugar is produced.

Questions 1-8.

1. The union of carbon dioxide and water to form starch results in an excess of

    A. hydrogen B. carbon C. oxygen
    D. carbon monoxide E. hydrogen peroxide

2. Synthesis of carbohydrates takes place

    A. in the stomata
    B. in the intercellular spaces of leaves
    C. in the walls of plant cells
    D. within the plasma membranes of plant cells
    E. within plant cells that contain chloroplasts

3. In the process of photosynthesis, chlorophyl acts as a

    A. carbohydrate B. source of carbon dioxide
    C. catalyst D. source of chemical energy
    E. plasma membrane

4. In which of the following places are there the GREATEST number of hours in which photosynthesis can take place during the month of December?

    A. Buenos Aires, Argentina B. Caracas, Venezuela
    C. Fairbanks, Alaska D. Quito, Ecuador
    E. Calcutta, India

5. During photosynthesis, molecules of carbon dioxide enter the stomata of leaves because

   A. the molecules are already in motion
   B. they are forced through the stomata by the son's rays
   C. chlorophyl attracts them
   D. a chemical change takes place in the stomata
   E. oxygen passes out through the stomata

6. Besides food manufacture, another USEFUL result of photosynthesis is that it

   A. aids in removing poisonous gases from the air
   B. helps to maintain the existing proportion of gases in the air
   C. changes complex compounds into simpler compounds
   D. changes certain waste products into hydrocarbons
   E. changes chlorophyl into useful substances

7. A process that is almost the exact reverse of photosynthesis is the

   A. rusting of iron
   B. burning of wood
   C. digestion of starch
   D. ripening of fruit
   E. storage of food in seeds

8. The leaf of the tomato plant will be unable to carry on photosynthesis if the

   A. upper surface of the leaf is coated with vaseline
   B. upper surface of the leaf is coated with lampblack
   C. lower surface of the leaf is coated with lard
   D. leaf is placed in an atmosphere of pure carbon dioxide
   E. entire leaf is coated with lime

TEST 2

DIRECTIONS: Each question or incomplete statement is followed by several suggested answers or completions. Select the one that BEST answers the question or completes the statement. *PRINT THE LETTER OF THE CORRECT ANSWER IN THE SPACE AT THE RIGHT.*

PASSAGE

The only carbohydrate which the human body can absorb and oxidize is the simple sugar glucose. Therefore, all carbohydrates which are consumed must be changed to glucose by the body before they can be used. There are specific enzymes in the mouth, the stomach, and the small intestine which break down complex carbohydrates. All the monosaccharides are changed to glucose by enzymes secreted by the intestinal glands, and the glucose is absorbed by the capillaries of the villi.

The following simple test is used to determine the presence of a reducing sugar. If Benedict's solution is added to a solution containing glucose or one of the other reducing sugars and the resulting mixture is heated, a brick-red precipitate will be formed. This test was carried out on several substances and the information in the following table was obtained. "P" indicates that the precipitate was formed and "N" indicates that no reaction was observed.

Material Tested	Observation
Crushed grapes in water	P
Cane sugar in water	N
Fructose	P
Molasses	N

Questions 1-2.

1. From the results of the test made upon crushed grapes in water, one may say that grapes contain

   A. glucose B. sucrose C. a reducing sugar
   D. no sucrose E. no glucose

2. Which one of the following foods probably undergoes the LEAST change during the process of carbohydrate digestion in the human body?

   A. Cane sugar B. Fructose C. Molasses
   D. Bread E. Potato

TEST 3

DIRECTIONS: Each question or incomplete statement is followed by several suggested answers or completions. Select the one that BEST answers the question or completes the statement. *PRINT THE LETTER OF THE CORRECT ANSWER IN THE SPACE AT THE RIGHT.*

PASSAGE

The British pressure suit was made in two pieces and joined around the middle in contrast to the other suits, which were one-piece suits with a removable helmet. Oxygen was supplied through a tube, and a container of soda lime absorbed carbon dioxide and water vapor. The pressure was adjusted to a maximum of 2 1/2 pounds per square inch (130 millimeters) higher than the surrounding air. Since pure oxygen was used, this produced a partial pressure of 130 millimeters, which is sufficient to sustain the flier at any altitude.

Using this pressure suit, the British established a world's altitude record of 49,944 feet in 1936 and succeeded in raising it to 53,937 feet the following year. The pressure suit is a compromise solution to the altitude problem. Full sea-level pressure can not be maintained, as the suit would be so rigid that the flier could not move arms or legs. Hence a pressure one third to one fifth that of sea level has been used. Because of these lower pressures, oxygen has been used to raise the partial pressure of alveolar oxygen to normal.

Questions 1-9.

1. The MAIN constituent of air not admitted to the pressure suit described was   1.__

   A. oxygen   B. nitrogen   C. water vapor
   D. carbon dioxide E. hydrogen

2. The pressure within the suit exceeded that of the surrounding air by an amount equal to 130 millimeters of   2.__

   A. mercury   B. water   C. air
   D. oxygen   E. carbon dioxide

3. The normal atmospheric pressure at sea level is   3.__

   A. 130 mm   B. 250 mm   C. 760 mm
   D. 1000 mm   E. 1300 mm

4. The water vapor that was absorbed by the soda lime came from   4.__

   A. condensation
   B. the union of oxygen with carbon dioxide
   C. body metabolism
   D. the air within the pressure suit
   E. water particles in the upper air

5. The HIGHEST altitude that has been reached with the British pressure suit is about   5.__

   A. 130 miles   B. 2 1/2 miles   C. 6 miles
   D. 10 miles   E. 5 miles

6. If the pressure suit should develop a leak, the

   A. oxygen supply would be cut off
   B. suit would fill up with air instead of oxygen
   C. pressure within the suit would drop to zero
   D. pressure within the suit would drop to that of the surrounding air
   E. suit would become so rigid that the flier would be unable to move arms or legs

7. The reason why oxygen helmets are unsatisfactory for use in efforts to set higher altitude records is that

   A. it is impossible to maintain a tight enough fit at the neck
   B. oxygen helmets are too heavy
   C. they do not conserve the heat of the body as pressure suits do
   D. if a parachute jump becomes necessary, it can not be made while such a helmet is being worn
   E. oxygen helmets are too rigid

8. The pressure suit is termed a compromise solution because

   A. it is not adequate for stratosphere flying
   B. aviators can not stand sea-level pressure at high altitudes
   C. some suits are made in two pieces, others in one
   D. other factors than maintenance of pressure have to be accommodated
   E. full atmospheric pressure can not be maintained at high altitudes

9. The passage implies that

   A. the air pressure at 49,944 feet is approximately the same as it is at 53,937 feet
   B. pressure cabin planes are not practical at extremely high altitudes
   C. a flier's oxygen requirement is approximately the same at high altitudes as it is at sea level
   D. one-piece pressure suits with removable helmets are unsafe
   E. a normal alveolar oxygen supply is maintained if the air pressure is between one third and one fifth that of sea level

TEST 4

DIRECTIONS: Each question or incomplete statement is followed by several suggested answers or completions. Select the one that BEST answers the question or completes the statement. *PRINT THE LETTER OF THE CORRECT ANSWER IN THE SPACE AT THE RIGHT.*

PASSAGE

Chemical investigations show that during muscle contraction the store of organic phosphates in the muscle fibers is altered as energy is released. In doing so, the organic phosphates (chiefly adenoisine triphosphate and phospho-creatine) are transformed anaerobically to organic compounds plus phosphates. As soon as the organic phosphates begin to break down in muscle contraction, the glycogen in the muscle fibers also transforms into lactic acid plus free energy; this energy the muscle fiber uses to return the organic compounds plus phosphates into high-energy organic phosphates ready for another contraction. In the presence of oxygen, the lactic acid from the glycogen decomposition is changed also. About one-fifth of it is oxidized to form water and carbon dioxide and to yield another supply of energy. This time the energy is used to transform the remaining four-fifths of the lactic acid into glycogen again.

Questions 1-5.

1. The energy for muscle contraction comes directly from the

   A. breakdown of lactic acid into glycogen
   B. resynthesis of adenosine triphosphate
   C. breakdown of glycogen into lactic acid
   D. oxidation of lactic acid
   E. breakdown of the organic phosphates

2. Lactic acid does NOT accumulate in a muscle that

   A. is in a state of lacking oxygen
   B. has an ample supply of oxygen
   C. is in a state of fatigue
   D. is repeatedly being stimulated
   E. has an ample supply of glycogen

3. The energy for the resynthesis of adenosine triphosphate and phospho-creatine comes from the

   A. oxidation of lactic acid
   B. synthesis of organic phosphates
   C. change from glycogen to lactic acid
   D. resynthesis of glycogen
   E. change from lactic acid to glycogen

4. The energy for the resynthesis of glycogen comes from the

   A. breakdown of organic phosphates
   B. resynthesis of organic phosphates
   C. change occurring in one-fifth of the lactic acid

D. change occurring in four-fifths of the lactic acid
E. change occurring in four-fifths of glycogen

5. The breakdown of the organic phosphates into organic compounds plus phosphates is an 5._____

   A. anobolic reaction   B. aerobic reaction
   C. endothermic reaction   D. exothermic reaction
   E. anaerobic reaction

TEST 5

DIRECTIONS: Each question or incomplete statement is followed by several suggested answers or completions. Select the one that BEST answers the question or completes the statement. *PRINT THE LETTER OF THE CORRECT ANSWER IN THE SPACE AT THE RIGHT.*

PASSAGE

And with respect to that theory of the origin of the forms of life peopling our globe, with which Darwin's name is bound up as closely as that of Newton with the theory of gravitation, nothing seems to be further from the mind of the present generation than any attempt to smother it with ridicule or to crush it by vehemence of denunciation. "The struggle for existence," and "natural selection," have become household words and everyday conceptions. The reality and the importance of the natural processes on which Darwin founds his deductions are no more doubted than those of growth and multiplication; and, whether the full potency attributed to them is admitted or not, no one is unmindful of or at all doubts their vast and far-reaching significance. Wherever the biological sciences are studied, the "Origin of Species" lights the path of the investigator; wherever they are taught it permeates the course of instruction. Nor has the influence of Darwinian ideas been less profound beyond the realms of biology. The oldest of all philosophies, that of evolution, was bound hand and foot and cast into utter darkness during the millennium of theological scholasticism. But Darwin poured new life-blood into the ancient frame; the bonds burst, and the revivified thought of ancient Greece has proved itself to be a more adequate expression of the universal order of things than any of the schemes which have been accepted by the credulity and welcomed by the superstition of seventy later generations of men.

Questions 1-7.

1. Darwin's theory of the origin of the species is based on

    A. theological deductions
    B. the theory of gravitation
    C. Greek mythology
    D. natural processes evident in the universe
    E. extensive reading in the biological sciences

2. The passage implies that

    A. thought in ancient Greece was dead
    B. the theory of evolution is now universally accepted
    C. the "Origin of Species" was seized by the Church
    D. Darwin was influenced by Newton
    E. the theories of "the struggle for existence" and "natural selection" are too evident to be scientific

3. The idea of evolution

    A. was suppressed for 1,000 years
    B. is falsely claimed by Darwin
    C. has swept aside all superstition
    D. was outworn even in ancient Greece
    E. has revolutionized the universe

4. The processes of growth and multiplication   4._____

    A. have been replaced by others discovered by Darwin
    B. were the basis for the theory of gravitation
    C. are "the struggle for existence" and "natural selection"
    D. are scientific theories not yet proved
    E. are accepted as fundamental processes of nature

5. Darwin's treatise on evolution   5._____

    A. traces life on the planets from the beginning of time to the present day
    B. was translated from the Greek
    C. contains an ancient philosophy in modern, scientific guise
    D. has had a profound effect on evolution
    E. has had little notice outside scientific circles

6. The theory of evolution   6._____

    A. was first advanced in the "Origin of Species"
    B. was suppressed by the ancient Greeks
    C. did not get beyond the monasteries during the millennium
    D. is philosophical, not scientific
    E. was elaborated and revived by Darwin

7. Darwin has contributed GREATLY toward   7._____

    A. a universal acceptance of the processes of nature
    B. reviving the Greek intellect
    C. ending the millennium of theological scholasticism
    D. a satisfactory explanation of scientific theory
    E. easing the struggle for existence

TEST 6

DIRECTIONS: Each question or incomplete statement is followed by several suggested answers or completions. Select the one that BEST answers the question or completes the statement. *PRINT THE LETTER OF THE CORRECT ANSWER IN THE SPACE AT THE RIGHT.*

PASSAGE

The higher forms of plants and animals, such as seed plants and vertebrates, are similar or alike in many respects but decidedly different in others. For example, both of these groups of organisms carry on digestion, respiration, reproduction, conduction, growth, and exhibit sensitivity to various stimuli. On the other hand, a number of basic differences are evident. Plants have no excretory systems comparable to those of animals. Plants have no heart or similar pumping organ. Plants are very limited in their movements. Plants have nothing similar to the animal nervous system. In addition, animals can not synthesize carbohydrates from inorganic substances. Animals do not have special regions of growth, comparable to terminal and lateral meristems in plants, which persist through-out the life span of the organism. And, finally, the animal cell "wall" is only a membrane, while plant cell walls are more rigid, usually thicker, and may be composed of such substances as cellulose, lignin, pectin, cutin, and suberin. These characteristics are important to an understanding of living organisms and their functions and should, consequently, be carefully considered in plant and animal studies

Questions 1-7.

1. Which of the following do animals lack?

    A. Ability to react to stimuli
    B. Ability to conduct substances from one place to another
    C. Reproduction by gametes
    D. A cell membrane
    E. A terminal growth region

2. Which of the following statements is false?

    A. Animal cell "walls" are composed of cellulose.
    B. Plants grow as long as they live.
    C. Plants produce sperms and eggs.
    D. All vertebrates have hearts.
    E. Wood is dead at maturity.

3. Respiration in plants takes place

    A. only during the day
    B. only in the presence of carbon dioxide
    C. both day and night
    D. only at night
    E. only in the presence of certain stimuli

4. An example of a vertebrate is the

    A. earthworm   B. starfish   C. amoeba
    D. cow   E. insect

1._

2._

3._

4._

5. Which of the following statements is true? 5.____

   A. All animals eat plants as a source of food.
   B. Respiration, in many ways, is the reverse of photo-synthesis.
   C. Man is an invertebrate animal.
   D. Since plants have no hearts, they can not develop high pressures in their cells.
   E. Plants can not move.

6. Which of the following do plants lack? 6.____

   A. A means of movement
   B. Pumping structures
   C. Special regions of growth
   D. Reproduction by gametes
   E. A digestive process

7. A substance that can be synthesized by green plants but NOT by animals is 7.____

   A. protein   B. cellulose   C. carbon dioxide
   D. uric acid   E. water

TEST 7

DIRECTIONS: Each question or incomplete statement is followed by several suggested answers or completions. Select the one that BEST answers the question or completes the statement. *PRINT THE LETTER OF THE CORRECT ANSWER IN THE SPACE AT THE RIGHT.*

PASSAGE

Sodium chloride, being by far the largest constituent of the mineral matter of the blood, assumes special significance in the regulation of water exchanges in the organism. And, as Cannon has emphasized repeatedly, these latter are more extensive and more important than may at first thought appear. He points out "there are a number of circulations of the fluid out of the body and back again, without loss." Thus, by example, it is estimated that from a quart and one-half of water daily "leaves the body" when it enters the mouth as saliva; another one or two quarts are passed out as gastric juice; and perhaps the same amount is contained in the bile and the secretions of the pancreas and the intestinal wall. This large volume of water enters the digestive processes; and practically all of it is reabsorbed through the intestinal wall, where it performs the equally important function of carrying in the digested foodstuffs. These and other instances of what Cannon calls "the conservative use of water in our bodies" involve essentially osmotic pressure relationships in which the concentration of sodium chloride plays an important part.

Questions 1-11.

1. This passage implies that

   A. the contents of the alimentary canal are not to be considered within the body
   B. sodium chloride does not actually enter the body
   C. every particle of water ingested is used over and over again
   D. water can not be absorbed by the body unless it contains sodium chloride
   E. substances can pass through the intestinal wall in only one direction

2. According to this passage, which of the following processes requires MOST water? The

   A. absorption of digested foods
   B. secretion of gastric juice
   C. secretion of saliva
   D. production of bile
   E. concentration of sodium chloride solution

3. A body fluid that is NOT saline is

   A. blood   B. urine   C. bile
   D. gastric juice E. saliva

4. An organ that functions as a storage reservoir from which large quantities of water are reabsorbed into the body is the

   A. kidney   B. liver   C. large intestine
   D. mouth   E. pancreas

334

5. Water is reabsorbed into the body by the process of

   A. secretion   B. excretion   C. digestion
   D. osmosis   E. oxidation

6. Digested food enters the body PRINCIPALLY through the

   A. mouth   B. liver   C. villi
   D. pancreas   E. stomach

7. The metallic element found in the blood in compound form and present there in larger quantities than any other metallic element is

   A. iron   B. calcium   C. magnesium
   D. chlorine   E. sodium

8. An organ that removes water from the body and prevents its reabsorption for use in the body processes is the

   A. pancreas   B. liver   C. small intestine
   D. lungs   E. large intestine

9. In which of the following processes is sodium chloride removed MOST rapidly from the body?

   A. Digestion   B. Breathing   C. Oxidation
   D. Respiration E. Perspiration

10. Which of the following liquids would pass from the alimentary canal into the blood MOST rapidly?

    A. A dilute solution of sodium chloride in water
    B. Gastric juice
    C. A concentrated solution of sodium chloride in water
    D. Digested food
    E. Distilled water

11. The reason why it is unsafe to drink ocean water even under conditions of extreme thirst is that it

    A. would reduce the salinity of the blood to a dangerous level
    B. contains dangerous disease germs
    C. contains poisonous salts
    D. would greatly increase the salinity of the blood
    E. would cause salt crystals to form in the blood stream

TEST 8

DIRECTIONS: Each question or incomplete statement is followed by several suggested answers or completions. Select the one that BEST answers the question or completes the statement. *PRINT THE LETTER OF THE CORRECT ANSWER IN THE SPACE AT THE RIGHT.*

PASSAGE

The discovery of antitoxin and its specific antagonistic effect upon toxin furnished an opportunity for the accurate investigation of the relationship of a bacterial antigen and its antibody. Toxin-antitoxin reactions were the first immunological processes to which experimental precision could be applied, and the discovery of principles of great importance resulted from such studies. A great deal of the work was done with diphtheria toxin and antitoxin and the facts elucidated with these materials are in principle applicable to similar substances.

The simplest assumption to account for the manner in which an antitoxin renders a toxin innocuous would be that the antitoxin destroys the toxin. Roux and Buchner, however, advanced the opinion that the antitoxin did not act directly upon the toxin, but affected it indirectly through the mediation of tissue cells. Ehrlich, on the other hand, conceived the reaction of toxin and antitoxin as a direct union, analogous to the chemical neutralization of an acid by a base.

The conception of toxin destruction was conclusively refuted by the experiments of Calmette. This observer, working with snake poison, found that the poison itself (unlike most other toxins) possessed the property of resisting heat to 100 degrees C, while its specific antitoxin, like other antitoxins, was destroyed at or about 70 degrees C. Nontoxic mixtures of the two substanues, when subjected to heat, regained their toxic properties. The natural inference from these observations was that the toxin in the original mixture had not been destroyed, but had been merely inactiviated by the presence of the antitoxin and again set free after destruction of the antitoxin by heat.

Questions 1-10.

1. Both toxins and antitoxins ORDINARILY

    A. are completely destroyed at body temperatures
    B. are extremely resistant to heat
    C. can exist only in combination
    D. are destroyed at 180° F
    E. are products of nonliving processes

2. MOST toxins can be destroyed by

    A. bacterial action B. salt solutions
    C. boiling D. diphtheria antitoxin
    E. other toxins

3. Very few disease organisms release a true toxin into the blood stream. It would follow, then, that

    A. studies of snake venom reactions have no value
    B. studies of toxin-antitoxin reactions are of little importance

C. the treatment of most diseases must depend upon information obtained from study of a few
D. antitoxin plays an important part in the body defense against the great majority of germs
E. only toxin producers are dangerous

4. A person becomes susceptible to infection again immediately after recovering from   4._____

   A. mumps   B. tetanus   C. diphtheria
   D. smallpox   E. tuberculosis

5. City people are more frequently immune to communicable diseases than country people are because   5._____

   A. country people eat better food
   B. city doctors are better than country doctors
   C. the air is more healthful in the country
   D. country people have fewer contacts with disease carriers
   E. there are more doctors in the city than in the country

6. The substances that provide us with immunity to disease are found in the body in the   6._____

   A. blood serum   B. gastric juice   C. urine
   D. white blood cells E. red blood cells

7. A person ill with diphtheria would MOST likely be treated with   7._____

   A. diphtheria toxin   B. diphtheria toxoid
   C. dead diphtheria germs   D. diphtheria antitoxin
   E. live diphtheria germs

8. To determine susceptibility to diphtheria, an individual may be given the   8._____

   A. Wassermann test   B. Schick test
   C. Widal test   D. Dick test
   E. Kahn test

9. Since few babies under six months of age contract diphtheria, young babies PROBABLY   9._____

   A. are never exposed to diphtheria germs
   B. have high body temperatures that destroy the toxin if acquired
   C. acquire immunity from their mothers
   D. acquire immunity from their fathers
   E. are too young to become infected

10. Calmette's findings   10._____

    A. contradicted both Roux and Buchner's opinion and Ehrlich's conception
    B. contradicted Roux and Buchner, but supported Ehrlich
    C. contradicted Ehrlich, but supported Roux and Buchner
    D. were consistent with both theories
    E. had no bearing on the point at issue

TEST 9

DIRECTIONS: Each question or incomplete statement is followed by several suggested answers or completions. Select the one that BEST answers the question or completes the statement. *PRINT THE LETTER OF THE CORRECT ANSWER IN THE SPACE AT THE RIGHT.*

PASSAGE

In the days of sailing ships, when voyages were long and uncertain, provisions for many months were stored without refrigeration in the holds of the ships. Naturally no fresh or perishable foods could be included. Toward the end of particularly long voyages the crews of such ships became ill and often many died from scurvy. Many men, both scientific and otherwise, tried to devise a cure for scurvy. Among the latter was John Hall, a son-in-law of William Shakespeare, who cured some cases of scurvy by administering a sour brew made from scurvy grass and water cress.

The next step was the suggestion of William Harvey that scurvy could be prevented by giving the men lemon juice. He thought that the beneficial substance was the acid contained in the fruit.

The third step was taken by Dr. James Lind, an English naval surgeon, who performed the following experiment with 12 sailors, all of whom were sick with scurvy: Each was given the same diet, except that four of the men received small amounts of dilute sulfuric acid, four others were given vinegar and the remaining four were given lemons. Only those who received the fruit recovered.

Questions 1-7.

1. Credit for solving the problem described above belongs to

   A. Hall, because he first devised a cure for scurvy
   B. Harvey, because he first proposed a solution of the problem
   C. Lind, because he proved the solution by means of an experiment
   D. both Harvey and Lind, because they found that lemons are more effective than scurvy grass or water cress
   E. all three men, because each made some contribution

2. A good substitute for lemons in the treatment of scurvy is

   A. fresh eggs   B. tomato juice   C. cod-liver oil
   D. liver   E. whole-wheat bread

3. The number of control groups that Dr. Lind used in his experiment was

   A. one   B. two   C. three   D. four   E. none

4. A substance that will turn blue litmus red is

   A. aniline   B. lye   C. ice
   D. vinegar   E. table salt

5. The hypothesis tested by Lind was:

   A. Lemons contain some substance not present in vinegar.
   B. Citric acid is the most effective treatment for scurvy.

C. Lemons contain some unknown acid that will cure scurvy.
D. Some specific substance, rather than acids in general, is needed to cure scurvy.
E. The substance needed to cure scurvy is found only in lemons.

6. A problem that Lind's experiment did NOT solve was: 6.____

   A. Will citric acid alone cure scurvy?
   B. Will lemons cure scurvy?
   C. Will either sulfuric acid or vinegar cure scurvy?
   D. Are all substances that contain acids equally effective as a treatment for scurvy?
   E. Are lemons more effective than either vinegar or sulfuric acid in the treatment of scurvy?

7. The PRIMARY purpose of a controlled scientific experiment is to 7.____

   A. get rid of superstitions
   B. prove a hypothesis is correct
   C. disprove a theory that is false
   D. determine whether a hypothesis is true or false
   E. discover new facts

TEST 10

DIRECTIONS: Each question or incomplete statement is followed by several suggested answers or completions. Select the one that BEST answers the question or completes the statement. *PRINT THE LETTER OF THE CORRECT ANSWER IN THE SPACE AT THE RIGHT.*

PASSAGE

The formed elements of the blood are the red corpuscles or erythrocytes, the white corpuscles or leucocytes, the blood platelets, and the so-called blood dust or hemoconiae. Together, these constitute 30-40 per cent by volume of the whole blood, the remainder being taken up by the plasma. In man, there are normally 5,000,000 red cells per cubic millimeter of blood; the count is somewhat lower in women. Variations occur frequently, especially after exercise or a heavy meal, or at high altitudes. Except in camels, which have elliptical corpuscles, the shape of the mammalian corpuscle is that of a circular, nonnucleated, bi-concave disk. The average diameter usually given is 7.7 microns, a value obtained by examining dried preparations of blood and considered by Ponder to be too low. Ponder's own observations, made on red cells in the fresh state, show the human corpuscle to have an average diameter of 8.8 microns. When circulating in the blood vessels, the red cell does not maintain a fixed shape but changes its form constantly, especially in the small capillaries. The red blood corpuscles are continually undergoing destruction, new corpuscles being formed to replace them. The average life of red corpuscles has been estimated by various investigators to be between three and six weeks. Preceding destruction, changes in the composition of the cells are believed to occur which render them less resistant. In the process of destruction, the lipids of the membrane are dissolved and the hemoglobin which is liberated is the most important, though probably not the only, source of bilirubin. The belief that the liver is the only site of red cell destruction is no longer generally held. The leucocytes, of which there are several forms, usually number between 7000 and 9000 per cubic millimeter of blood. These increase in number in disease, particularly when there is bacterial infection.

Questions 1-10.

1. Leukemia is a disease involving the

   A. red cells   B. white cells   C. plasma
   D. blood platelets   E. blood dust

2. Are the erythrocytes in the blood increased in number after a heavy meal? The paragraph implies that this

   A. is true   B. holds only for camels
   C. is not true   D. may be true
   E. depends on the number of white cells

3. When blood is dried, the red cells

   A. contract   B. remain the same size   C. disintegrate
   D. expand   E. become elliptical

4. Ponder is probably classified as a professional

   A. pharmacist   B. physicist   C. psychologist
   D. physiologist   E. psychiatrist

5. The term "erythema" when applied to skin conditions signifies

   A. redness
   B. swelling
   C. irritation
   D. pain
   E. roughness

6. Lipids are insoluble in water and soluble in such solvents as ether, chloroform and benzene. It may be inferred that the membranes of red cells MOST closely resemble

   A. egg white
   B. sugar
   C. bone
   D. butter
   E. cotton fiber

7. Analysis of a sample of blood yields cell counts of 4,800,000 erythrocytes and 16,000 leucocytes per cubic millimeter. These data suggest that the patient from whom the blood was taken

   A. is anemic
   B. has been injuriously invaded by germs
   C. has been exposed to high-pressure air
   D. has a normal cell count
   E. has lost a great deal of blood

8. Bilirubin, a bile pigment, is

   A. an end product of several different reactions
   B. formed only in the liver
   C. formed from the remnants of the cell membranes of erythrocytes
   D. derived from hemoglobin exclusively
   E. a precursor of hemoglobin

9. Bancroft found that the blood count of the natives in the Peruvian Andes differed from that usually accepted as normal. The blood PROBABLY differed in respect to

   A. leucocytes
   B. blood platelets
   C. cell shapes
   D. erythrocytes
   E. hemoconiae

10. Hemoglobin is probably NEVER found

    A. free in the blood stream
    B. in the red cells
    C. in women's blood
    D. in the blood after exercise
    E. in the leucocytes

TEST 11

Questions 1-7.

DIRECTIONS: Each question or incomplete statement is followed by several suggested answers or completions. Select the one that BEST answers the question or completes the statement. *PRINT THE LETTER OF THE CORRECT ANSWER IN THE SPACE AT THE RIGHT.*

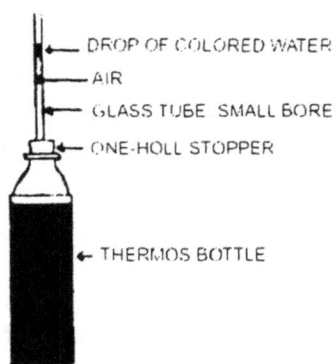

1. The device shown in the diagram above indicates changes that are measured more accurately by a(n)

   A. thermometer B. hygrometer C. anemometer
   D. hydrometer   E. barometer

   1.___

2. If the device is placed in a cold refrigerator for 72 hours, which of the following is MOST likely to happen?

   A. The stopper will be forced out of the bottle.
   B. The drop of water will evaporate.
   C. The drop will move downward.
   D. The drop will move upward.
   E. No change will take place.

   2.___

3. When the device was carried in an elevator from the first floor to the sixth floor of a building, the drop of colored water moved about 1/4 inch in the tube. Which of the following is MOST probably true? The drop moved

   A. *downward* because there was a decrease in the air pressure
   B. *upward* because there was a decrease in the air pressure
   C. *downward* because there was an increase in the air temperature
   D. *upward* because there was an increase in the air temperature
   E. *downward* because there was an increase in the temperature and a decrease in the pressure

   3.___

4. The part of a thermos bottle into which liquids are poured consists of

   A. a single-walled, metal flask coated with silver
   B. two flasks, one of glass and one of silvered metal
   C. two silvered-glass flasks separated by a vacuum
   D. two silver flasks separated by a vacuum
   E. a single-walled, glass flask with a silver-colored coating

   4.___

342

5. The thermos bottle is MOST similar in principle to

   A. the freezing unit in an electric refrigerator
   B. radiant heaters
   C. solar heating systems
   D. storm windows
   E. a thermostatically controlled heating system

6. In a plane flying at an altitude where the air pressure is only half the normal pressure at sea level, the plane's altimeter should read, *approximately,*

   A. 3000 feet   B. 9000 feet   C. 18000 feet
   D. 27000 feet   E. 60000 feet

7. Which of the following is the POOREST conductor of heat?

   A. Air under a pressure of 1.5 pounds per square inch
   B. Air under a pressure of 15 pounds per square inch
   C. Unsilvered glass
   D. Silvered glass
   E. Silver

TEST 12

DIRECTIONS: Each question or incomplete statement is followed by several suggested answers or completions. Select the one that BEST answers the question or completes the statement. *PRINT THE LETTER OF THE CORRECT ANSWER IN THE SPACE AT THE RIGHT.*

PASSAGE

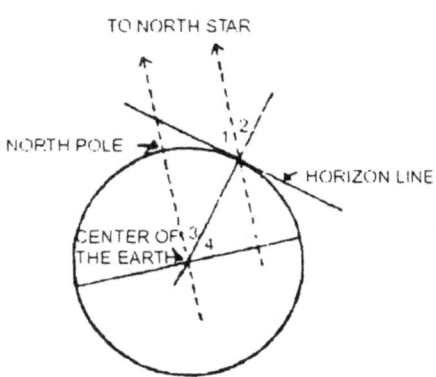

The latitude of any point on the earth's surface is the angle between a plumb line dropped to the center of the earth from that point and the plane of the earth's equator. Since it is impossible to go to the center of the earth to measure latitude, the latitude of any point may be determined indirectly as shown in the accompanying diagram.

It will be recalled that the axis of the earth, if extended out-ward, passes very near the North Star. Since the North Star is, for all practical purposes, infinitely distant, the line of sight to the North Star of an observer on the surface of the earth is virtually parallel with the earth's axis. Angle 1, then, in the diagram represents the angular distance of the North Star above the horizon. Angle 2 is equal to angle 3, because when two parallel lines are intersected by a straight line, the corresponding angles are equal. Angle 1 plus angle 2 is a right angle and so is angle 3 plus angle 4. Therefore, angle 1 equals angle 4 because when equals are subtracted from equals the results are equal.

Questions 1-10.

1. If an observer finds that the angular distance of the North Star above the horizon is 30, his latitude is

    A. 15° N   B. 30° N   C. 60° N   D. 90° N   E. 120° N

2. To an observer on the equator, the North Star would be

    A. 30° above the horizon   B. 60° above the horizon
    C. 90° above the horizon   D. on the horizon
    E. below the horizon

3. To an observer on the Arctic Circle, the North Star would be   3.____

   A. directly overhead
   B. 23 1/2° above the horizon
   C. 66 1/2° above the horizon
   D. on the horizon
   E. below the horizon

4. The distance around the earth along a certain parallel of latitude is 3600 miles. At that latitude, how many miles are there in one degree of longitude?   4.____

   A. 1 mile   B. 10 miles   C. 30 miles
   D. 69 miles   E. 100 miles

5. At which of the following latitudes would the sun be DIRECTLY overhead at noon on June 21?   5.____

   A. 0°   B. 23 1/2°S   C. 23 1/2°N
   D. 66 1/2°N   E. 66 1/2°S

6. On March 21 the number of hours of daylight at places on the Arctic Circle is   6.____

   A. none   B. 8   C. 12   D. 16   E. 24

7. The distance from the equator to the 45th parallel, measured along a meridian, is, *approximately,*   7.____

   A. 450 miles   B. 900 miles   C. 1250 miles
   D. 3125 miles   E. 6250 miles

8. The difference in time between the meridians that pass through longitude 45°E and longitude 105°W   8.____

   A. 6 hours   B. 2 hours   C. 8 hours
   D. 4 hours   E. 10 hours

9. Which of the following is NOT a great circle or part of a great circle?   9.____

   A. Arctic Circle
   B. 100th meridian
   C. Equator
   D. Shortest distance between New York and London
   E. Greenwich meridian

10. At which of the following places does the sun set EARLIEST on June 21?   10.____

    A. Montreal, Canada   B. Santiago, Chile
    C. Mexico City, Mexico   D. Lima, Peru
    E. Manila, P.I.

KEY (CORRECT ANSWERS)

TEST 1		**TEST 2**		**TEST 3**		**TEST 4**	
1. C	5. A	1. C		1. B	6. D	1. A	
2. E	6. B	2. B		2. A	7. D	2. B	
3. C	7. B			3. C	8. E	3. C	
4. A	8. C			4. C	9. C	4. C	
				5. D		5. D	

TEST 5		**TEST 6**		**TEST 7**		**TEST 8**	
1. D	5. D	1. E	5. B	1. A	6. C	1. D	6. A
2. B	6. E	2. A	6. B	2. A	7. E	2. C	7. D
3. A	7. A	3. C	7. B	3. D	8. D	3. C	8. B
4. E		4. D		4. C	9. E	4. E	9. C
				5. D	10. E	5. D	10. D
					11. D		

TEST 9		**TEST 10**		**TEST 11**		**TEST 12**	
1. E	5. D	1. B	6. D	1. A	5. D	1. B	6. C
2. B	6. A	2. D	7. B	2. C	6. C	2. D	7. D
3. B	7. D	3. A	8. A	3. B	7. A	3. C	8. E
4. D		4. D	9. D	4. C		4. B	9. A
		5. A	10. E			5. C	10. B

www.ingramcontent.com/pod-product-compliance
Lightning Source LLC
Chambersburg PA
CBHW081757300426
44116CB00014B/2153